Evidence-Based
Practice for Nurses

Evidence-Based Practice for Nurses

Janet Barker

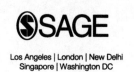

Los Angeles | London | New Delhi
Singapore | Washington DC

First published 2010
Reprinted 2010

SAGE Publications Ltd
1 Oliver's Yard
55 City Road
London EC1Y 1SP

SAGE Publications Inc.
2455 Teller Road
Thousand Oaks, California 91320

SAGE Publications India Pvt Ltd
B 1/I 1 Mohan Cooperative Industrial Area
Mathura Road
New Delhi 110 044

SAGE Publications Asia-Pacific Pte Ltd
33 Pekin Street #02-01
Far East Square
Singapore 048763

Library of Congress Control Number: 2009927727

British Library Cataloguing in Publication data

A catalogue record for this book is available from the British Library

ISBN 978-1-84787-278-4
ISBN 978-1-84787-279-1 (pbk)

Typeset by C&M Digitals (P) Ltd, Chennai, India
Printed in Great Britain by the MPG Books Group
Printed on paper from sustainable resources

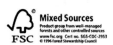

Mixed Sources
Product group from well-managed
forests and other controlled sources
www.fsc.org Cert no. SGS-COC-2953
© 1996 Forest Stewardship Council
FSC

Contents

Preface

EBP is seen as an essential component of nursing. The Nursing and Midwifery Council (NMC) (2008) identifies that registered nurses 'must deliver care based on best evidence or best practice.' Pearson et al (2008) identify that whatever position you hold in nursing – student or registered nurse; staff nurse or service manager – you are expected to be able to assess the quality of evidence used in practice and deliver care supported by best evidence. However, as you will see in the following chapters, there is a great deal of debate surrounding evidence-based practice (EBP) and what it means in reality for nursing and the delivery/management of care.

There are various skills and knowledge bases which you need to develop if you are to meet the NMC requirements; the challenges of modern practice; and fulfil your responsibilities as an accountable practitioner. The intention here is to provide you with a resource to help you navigate the process of EBP, develop the necessary knowledge and skills, and ensure your practice is based on best evidence.

There are a number of ways you can use this book. If you are new to the concept of EBP you may want to work through the chapters at your own pace and gain the necessary knowledge and skills in a step by step way. If you already have some insight into EBP, you may want to dip into various chapters as appropriate to your learning needs. Each chapter begins with a list of learning outcomes so you can identify what you should know at the end of it and ends with a summary of the main points, suggestions for further reading and useful e-resources. Key terms are highlighted and definitions given in the glossary.

What's in the book

The book falls into three sections, section one looks at the critical elements of EBP – evidence, clinical expertise, patient preference, local context - and how to find evidence. Chapter 1 considers what EBP is and why it is important that nurses understand and develop the necessary knowledge and skills. Chapter 2 explores issues in relation to what knowledge is and where it comes from; what knowledge is seen as underpinning the practice of nursing; what counts as good and appropriate evidence; and how to identify what it is that you want to know. Chapter 3 discusses issues related to clinical judgement, expertise and decision making. Issues related to patient preferences and local context are also addressed. Chapter 4 considers how you go about finding the evidence and developing a search strategy.

Section 2 provides an opportunity to explore the knowledge and skills associated with the critical appraisal of evidence, beginning with chapter 5, which identifies what is meant by critical appraisal and its role in the EBP process. Chapters 6 and 7 look at critical appraisal specifically in relation to quantitative and qualitative research respectively. Chapter 8 considers issues related to systematic review and its place in EBP. Critical appraisal tools to help with this process are provide in the appendices.

Finally, section 3 looks at how to make changes to practice once you have found and critically appraised the evidence. Chapter 9 considers how you integrate evidence into your own practice and how you can begin to influence change generally and help develop an EBP culture in the practice setting. Chapter 10 discusses issues related to your professional development, and how you ensure your practice continues to be evidence-based through the use of reflection and portfolio work. Templates for activities are provided in the appendices. Each section ends with a quiz to enable you to test your learning so far. At various points activities are used to help you develop your skills in certain areas. To help you consolidate your learning in relation to the issues discussed, each chapter ends with an EBP activity.

I hope you will find the book a useful resource, one that helps you to develop the knowledge and skills needed to ensure patients receive the best care possible – based on good evidence and aimed at achieving positive outcomes.

Part I
Introducing Evidence-Based Practice

1

Introduction: What is Evidence-Based Practice?

Learning Outcomes

By the end of the chapter you will be able to:

- define evidence-based practice;
- understand how evidence-based practice came into being;
- discuss the pros and cons of evidence-based practice;
- identify the components of evidence-based practice and the skills associated with it;
- consider why your practice needs to be evidence-based.

Introduction

Many terms are used in relation to evidence-based practice (EBP) – evidence-based nursing, evidence-based nursing practice, evidence-based medicine, evidence-based mental health and evidence-based health care. The idea of EBP is at the forefront of health-care discussions, leading Rycroft-Malone et al. to suggest that it has become a global phenomenon, with **evidence** being something of a 'buzz word' and rapidly becoming 'one of the most fashionable words in healthcare' (2004a: 82). A simple search of the CINAHL database, using the phrase '*evidence-based practice*', and limited to '*nursing*', revealed 3011 relevant articles. From this alone it is safe to say there has been an explosion of interest in this area.

Implicit in such discussions is the message that health care, wherever it is delivered, must be based on good, sound **evidence**. In days gone by, when asked why something was done in a particular way, a nurse's mantra was 'Sister says so' or 'We've always done it this way.' This is no longer sufficient and there is an expectation that strong evidence must underpin nurses' practice. Mantzoukas (2007) has identified that EBP is central to the notion of best practice, nurse accountability, and the need to ensure that nursing activities are transparent and safe.

Whilst the importance of research in the delivery of nursing care has always been emphasized, the idea of evidence-based practice is seen as focusing the minds of those involved in care delivery on the use of appropriate evidence.

There is also a perceived lack of enthusiasm in relation to the implementation of nursing research. Glasziou and Haynes (2005) proposed that some research, essential to the delivery of quality of care, will go unrecognized for years and suggested the major barriers to using evidence are time, effort and the skills involved in accessing information from the myriad of data available. EBP is seen as a way of addressing this.

Ingersoll (2000) has also argued that focusing EBP on care delivery reflects the differences between it and research. Research concentrates on knowledge discovery whereas in EBP the application of knowledge is central. In addition she has suggested that whilst this emphasis on EBP is a welcome initiative, the wholesale 'lifting' of approaches and methodologies from another discipline such as medicine is not. Nurses need to make sure that the evidence used is relevant to the practice of nursing. There is a range of such evidence that can inform practice – personal experience and reflection literature, research, policy, guidelines, clinical expertise, and audit (Dale, 2005) – all of which has its place within EBP and will be explored further in the various chapters of this book.

So what is EBP?

At its simplest, EBP is about good practice and improving the quality of care, however achieving this is a complex undertaking. Various definitions are available (see Box 1.1). French (1999) has suggested that there are certain key features of EBP, proposing it is:

- based on problems identified from the practitioner's area of practice;
- a combining of best evidence and professional expertise and an integration of this into current practice;
- about ensuring patients receive quality care, being part of quality improvement processes;
- about collaboration and requires a team approach.

Box 1.1   Definitions of EBP

RCN (1996: 3): 'Doing the right thing in the right way for the right patient at the right time'.

Flemming and Cullum (1997: 28): 'Evidence based health care involves using a combination of clinical expertise and best available evidence, together with patient preferences to inform decision making'.

Ingersoll (2000: 152): 'The conscientious, explicit and judicious use of theory-derived, research-based information in making decisions about care delivery to individuals or groups of patients and in consideration of individual needs and preferences'.

Dale (2005: 49): EBP involves 'the nurse making conscious judgements about available evidence'.

Cullen et al. (2008: 2): Evidence-based nursing is 'the application of valid, relevant, research-based information in nurse decision making'.

Considering the various definitions and French's key features it is fair to say that the critical elements of EBP can be represented as:

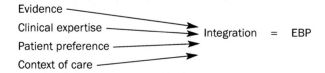

Where did the idea of EBP come from?

Professor Archie Cochrane, a British epidemiologist, is most frequently credited with starting the EBP movement. In his book *Effectiveness and Efficiency: Random Reflections on the Health Services* (Cochrane, 1972) he criticized the medical profession for not using appropriate evidence to guide and direct medical practice and challenged medicine to produce an evidence base. He argued there was a need to ensure treatment was delivered in the most effective way and to ensure that available evidence was used in a consistent way.

When Cochrane talked of evidence, he meant Randomised Control Trials (RCTs), which he viewed as providing the most reliable evidence on which to base medical care. RCTs are a form of research which used experimental designs to identify the effectiveness of interventions. The use of systematic reviews, which summarized the findings of a number of RCTs looking at similar areas of interest, was suggested as the 'gold standard' of the scientific evidence on which to base medical interventions.

The medical profession responded to Cochrane's challenge by creating the Cochrane Centre for systematic reviews, which opened in 1992 in Oxford. The Cochrane Collaboration was founded in 1993, consisting of international review groups (currently encompassing more than 11,500 people in 90 countries) covering a range of clinical areas and producing systematic reviews. These reviews are published electronically, updated regularly and there are now over 3000 of these available.

ACTIVITY

Visit the Cochrane Collaboration Website (http://www.cochrane.org) and identify one systematic review abstract that would be of interest in relation to your current clinical environment.

Other collaborations have emerged since this time. For example, the Joanna Briggs Institute (JBI) – an international EBP collaboration – was established in Australia in 1996. Its aim is to evaluate evidence from a wide range of sources, including all research methodologies, clinical experience and expertise. The JBI has identified three activities central to its role in relation to EBP:

- evidence synthesis – the bringing together of evidence in the form of systematic reviews;
- evidence transfer – targeting the evidence at clinical areas in forms that are easily accessible, such as 'best practice' information;
- evidence utilization – providing tools that will enable evidence to be used and embedded in practice, such as audit tools.

ACTIVITY

Visit the JBI website (http://joannabriggs.edu.au) and find a best practice sheet relevant to your most recent practice experience. Using this consider what implications this might have for your own clinical practice.

The idea for **evidence-based medicine** (EBM) grew out of Cochrane's work. McMaster Medical School in Canada is credited with coining the term in 1980 to describe a particular learning approach used in the school. This approach had four steps – formulating a question related to a clinical problem; searching the literature for relevant information; critically appraising the literature; and using the findings to direct clinical practice (Peile, 2004).

Sackett et al. (1996: 71) defined evidence-based medicine as 'the conscientious, explicit and judicious use of current best evidence in making decisions about the care of individual patients'. Whilst the underpinning principles of EBM were hotly debated, the medical profession in general began to accept the idea, and 1995 saw the first issue of the journal *Evidence-Based Medicine for Primary Care and Internal Medicine*, published by the British Medical Journal Group. Nursing, emulating its medical colleagues, began to explore the notion of basing their practice on reliable sources of evidence, which resulted in the journal *Evidence-Based Nursing* appearing in 1998. The Centre for Evidence-Based Nursing (CEBN) was also established at the University of York in 1998 (www.york.ac.uk/healthsciences/centres/evidence/cebn), with the aim of promoting evidence-based nursing through research, education and development.

Social and political drivers of EBP

Kitson (2002) suggests a number of factors facilitated the emergence of the emphasis on evidence at this time. The availability of 'knowledge' via the internet and other sources brought into being 'expert patients' – well educated and informed individuals who accessed information relating to health and illness. The

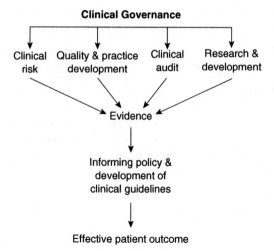

Figure 1.1   *Representation of the elements of clinical governance*

expectations of these expert patients were that health-care professions would be aware of and use up-to-date information/research in their delivery of care and treatment. There was no longer a willingness simply to accept treatment or care purely on the advice of a doctor or nurses.

The concept of EBP was also seen as attractive by government and NHS administrators because of its potential to provide cost effective care that was also seen as clinically effective (French, 1999). In the mid-1990s the government of the day identified that quality assurance was to be placed at the forefront of the NHS agenda. Two White Papers – *The New NHS: Modern and Dependable* (DoH, 1997) and *A First Class Service: Quality in the New NHS* (DoH, 1998) – outlined the plans for promoting **clinical effectiveness** and introducing **clinical governance**: these gave systems to ensure quality improvement mechanisms were adopted at all levels of health-care provision. Central to clinical governance were concepts of risk management and promoting clinical excellence. (See Figure 1.1 for an outline of the clinical governance framework.)

Clinical effectiveness is defined by the DoH (1998) as 'the extent to which specific clinical interventions when deployed in the field for a particular patient or population, do what they are intended to do, that is maintain and improve health and secure the greatest possible health gain'. The Department of Health also suggested the various stages to this process:

- the development of best practice guidelines;
- the transfer of knowledge into practice through education, audit and practice development;
- the evaluation of the impact of guidelines through audit and patient feedback.

Put simply, clinical effectiveness can be seen as identifying appropriate evidence in the form of research, clinical guidelines, systematic reviews and national standards; changing practice to include this evidence; evaluating the impact of any

Table 1.1   *Research, audit and service evaluation (adapted from Defining Research produced by the National Research Ethics Service, 2007)*

Research	Clinical audit	Service evaluations/patient feedback
Generates new knowledge	Generates information to promote effective care	Provides insight into current care
Tests hypotheses or generates theories	Identifies if care is of the required standard	Identifies what standard of care is delivered
Has clearly defined questions, aims and objectives	Measures care against an identified standard	Identifies the standard of care
Compares interventions/ activities and/or experiences of people	Measures an activity	Measures an activity
Collects and analyzes data relevant to the research question – this may or may not be data routinely collected	Collects and analyzes existing data relevant to the topic	Collects and analyzes existing data relevant to the topic
Has a clearly defined framework for sampling the population of interest	Population of interest are those who have been involved in the activity	Population of interest are those who have been involved in the activity

change and making the necessary adjustments through the use of clinical audit and patient feedback/service evaluation. Table 1.1 provides an overview of the key aspects of research – **clinical audit** and **service evaluation**.

Two organizations were created aimed at promoting an evidence-based approach to health care, which are known today as the National Institute of Health and Clinical Excellence (NICE) and the Healthcare Commission (HCC). These bodies provide guidance for health-care managers and practitioners and are charged with ensuring this guidance is followed in England and Wales. In Scotland the Health Technology Board fulfils a similar purpose. Clinical governance was introduced to ensure health care was both efficient and effective; health-care professionals were expected to show EBP supported all aspects of care delivery and service developments. It was hoped that the introduction of these measures would result in a shift in organizational culture from one that was reactive, responding as issues arise, to one with a proactive ethos, where the health care offered is known to be effective and therefore avoids unforeseen outcomes.

Concerns about EBP

Evidence-based approaches are not without their problems. Melnyk and Fineout–Overholt (2005) suggested that EBP is viewed by many as simply another term for research utilization. It has also been argued elsewhere that the value of research has been over-emphasized to the detriment of clinical judgement and person-centred approaches, while others point to a lack of evidence to support the notion that evidence-based practice improves health outcomes.

Kitson (2002) has pointed to an inherent tension between EBP and person-centred approaches. She has argued that clinical expertise is vital in ensuring that patients' experiences and needs are not sidelined in the pursuit of 'best evidence' in the form of research findings and the development of generalized clinical guidelines. Some individuals have suggested that such broad general principles are not applicable to certain aspects of care. Melnyk and Fineout-Overholt (2005) have identified this as a 'cookbook' approach, where a general recipe is followed with no consideration for the specific needs or preferences of individuals. There are concerns also around the ability to have a consensus in relation to the various interpretations available when translating evidence into guidelines and the relevance of these for individual areas of practice. There are also issues related to the updating of evidence and the ability to ensure that the information gathered is current. However, DiCenso et al. (2008) argue that as clinical expertise and decision-making processes are central to EBP, in considering the use of general guidelines both of these processes must be used in the same way with any form of evidence including guidance.

However Brady and Lewin (2007) identify that whilst the idea of clinical expertise is readily accepted by most experienced nurses, the majority of those same nurses are often unaware of the latest research in their area of practice. Nurses are generally presented as relying on intuition, tradition, and local policies/procedures to guide their practice. Stevens (2004) proposed that health-care providers will frequently not use current knowledge for a number of reasons, not least of these being the rapidly growing and changing body of research, some of which is difficult to apply to practice directly. As the aim of EBP is to deliver high quality care, nurses need to have an understanding of what the exact elements of EBP are and to then develop the necessary skills and knowledge to enable them to carry this out.

French (1999) suggested that as EBP is so closely linked with EBM and its preference for certain types of evidence, there is a danger that this promotes the use of medical knowledge over other forms and therefore leads to a medicalization of health-care environments to the detriment of other disciplines. Best evidence in the medical context is often taken to mean quantitative research findings – as identified above in the form of RCTs. Some have questioned its compatibility with nursing and the other health professions, suggesting instead the use of a more open approach. Dale (2005) proposed that this issue has the potential to create interprofessional conflict, as that what nursing may count as appropriate evidence on which to base practice may be somewhat different from that of the medical profession.

What skills are needed?

EBP is often represented as a process that has a number of steps within it. Sackett et al. (2000) have suggested a four-step model:

1. Ask an answerable question.
2. Find the appropriate evidence.
3. Critically appraise that evidence.
4. Apply the evidence to the patient, giving consideration to the individual needs, presentation and context.

The JBI has a similar model containing six steps (see Box 1.2).

Box 1.2   JBI model of EBP

- Search for evidence.
- Appraise evidence.
- Summarize evidence.
- Utilize.
- Embed.
- Evaluate the impact.

Stevens (2004) has also proposed a model to explain the stages of converting knowledge into meaningful evidence to be used in EBP. The Star Model of Knowledge Transformation takes the form of a five-point star with one of the stages of transformation (discovery, summary, translation, integration and evaluation) placed on each point. (See Table 1.2 for an overview of the stages.)

There are common themes that run through all these models which would suggest there is a need to develop particular skills and knowledge related to:

- the ability to identify what counts as appropriate evidence;
- forming a question to enable you to find evidence for consideration;
- developing a search strategy;
- finding the evidence;
- critically appraising the evidence;
- drawing on clinical expertise;
- issues concerned with patient preference;
- application to the context of care delivery;
- putting the evidence into practice.

Table 1.2   *ACE Star Model of Knowledge Translation (Stevens, 2004)*

Stage	Explanation.
Discovery	Generation of knowledge through scientific enquiry and primary research.
Summary	The bringing together of a body of research into a meaningful statement, usually in the form of a systematic review. This may also generate new knowledge through the combining of findings.
	This is seen as the first step of EBP.
Translation	Translation into relevant practice recommendations in the form of practice guidelines.
Integration	Individual and/or organization practices are changed.
Evaluation	Impact on health outcomes, satisfaction and efficiency is evaluated.

Why does your practice need to be evidence-based?

As Craig and Pearson (2007) have already identified, few in the health-care professions would disagree with the ideas underpinning EBP – namely, that care should be of the highest standard and delivered in the most effective way. Indeed practising without any 'evidence' to guide our actions amounts to little more than providing care that is based on trial and error, which none of us would advocate. However, as identified above, care is not always based on the best evidence, with Greenhalgh (2006) suggesting that many of the decisions made in health care are based on four main sources of information:

1. *Anecdotal information*   Here it is considered that 'it worked in situation X so it must be appropriate to (the similar) situation Y'. However, as Greenhalgh points out, while situations may seem very similar, patient responses are often very different.
2. *Press cuttings information*   Here changes are made to practice in response to reading one article or editorial, without critically appraising and considering the applicability of those results to the specific setting.
3. *Consensus statements*   Here a group of 'experts' will identify the best approaches based on their experiences/beliefs. Whilst clinical expertise does have a place in EBP, it does not operate without some problems. For example, clinical wisdom once held (and to a certain extent still does hold) that bed rest was the most appropriate form of treatment for acute lower back pain. However, research in 1986 demonstrated that this is potentially harmful.
4. *Cost minimization*   Here the limited resources available within a health-care setting will often result in choosing the cheapest option in an effort to spread resources as widely as possible. However, EBP can ensure the most effective use of limited and pressurised resources. Whilst certain types of care may appear more expensive on the surface, if these prove more effective, they may turn out to be cheaper in the long run.

Perhaps part of the problem related to nursing developing an EBP ethos is that nursing is often considered as more of an art than a science and as such certain types of evidence are valued above others, such as expert opinion and practice experience. However, Polit and Beck (2008: 4) identified that any nursing action must be 'clinically appropriate, cost effective and result in a positive outcome for clients'. The complexity of health care, and the uncertainty of people's responses to and experiences of different types of interventions, require that a full consideration is given to all the available evidence.

Patients are likely to know a great deal about their own health needs and to expect health professionals to base care decisions on the most up-to-date and clinically relevant information. There is also an expectation that professionals will be able to comment in an informed way on any research reported in the media and identify its relevance to and appropriateness for an individual's health needs. Miller and Forrest (2001) proposed that the ability to ensure that a professional's knowledge and skills remain current increases their professional credibility; allows them to be an important source of information to those in their care as well as colleagues; and enables all professionals involved in care delivery to make well informed decisions. It has also been suggested that EBP provides the framework by which such demands may be met and can foster a lifelong learning approach – an essential requirement in the health professions if staff are to remain effective in rapidly changing health–care environments.

EBP ACTIVITY

Consider the list of skills identified above as associated with EBP (listed on p. 10). Choose three areas which you feel you have most difficulty with and undertake a SWOT analysis in relation to each one using the grid in Appendix 1.

SUMMARY

- EBP is a global phenomenon which promotes the idea of best practice, clinical effectiveness and quality care and involves an integration of evidence, clinical expertise, patient preferences and the clinical context of care delivery to inform clinical decision making.
- EBP focuses on critically appraising evidence to support care delivery rather than research to discover new knowledge.
- The emergence of the expert patient has given rise to the need for health professionals to ensure they are up to date and their care is based on the best evidence available.
- Government initiatives have promoted EBP as a way of providing both clinically effective and cost effective health care.
- Various steps are associated with the EBP process – forming a question, finding evidence, critically appraising the evidence, integrating evidence into practice.
- The knowledge and skills associated with EPA are an essential component of nursing practice.

Further reading

Cranston, M. (2002) 'Clinical effectiveness and evidence-based practice', *Nursing Standard*, 16 (24): 39–43. This provides a concise account of the meaning of clinical governance, the place of clinical effectiveness within this concept, and the drive towards EBP.

Rycroft-Malone, J., Seers, K., Titchen, A., Harvey, G., Kitson, A. and McCormack, B. (2004) 'What counts as evidence in evidence-based practice?', *Journal of Advanced Nursing*, 47 (1): 81–90. This article gives a clear overview of the evidence-based movement and issues related to the nature of evidence.

Sackett, D.L., Rosenberg, W.M.C., Grey, J.A.M., Haynes, R.B. and Richardson, W.S. (1996) 'Evidence based medicine: what it is and what it isn't. It's about integrating individual clinical expertise and the best external evidence', *British Medical Journal*, 312 (7023): 71–2. Sackett et al. provide an explanation of the development of EBM and its key components, giving an insight into the beginnings of EBP.

E-resources

Centre for Evidence-Based Nursing: aims to promote evidence-based nursing through education, research and development.
www.york.ac.uk/healthsciences/centres/evidence/cebn

Cochrane Collaboration: promotes, supports and prepares systematic reviews, mainly in relation to effectiveness.
www.cochrane.org

Joanna Briggs Institute: promotes evidence-based health care through systematic reviews and a range of resources aimed at promoting evidence synthesis, transfer and utilization.
www.joannabriggs.edu.au

2

The Nature of Knowledge, Evidence and How to Ask the Right Questions

Learning Outcomes

By the end of the chapter you will be able to:

- discuss the nature of knowledge;
- identify what is meant by 'evidence';
- form a question to allow the identification and selection of best evidence;
- understand the use of the PICO framework in forming research questions.

Introduction

It is suggested that humans have a basic need for knowledge and thirst to know how things work and why things happen. Parahoo (1997) proposed that knowledge is essential for human survival, and central to decision making about daily life and achieving change in both people and the environment they live in. Prior to the eighteenth century much of people's understanding of the world and how it worked was based on beliefs related to superstitions and organized religions. However, the eighteenth century ushered in what we know as the era of 'Enlightenment' and the 'Age of Reason' which promoted different ways of thinking and knowing the world. The work of individuals known as 'encyclopedists' (generally leading philosophers of the day) and the publication of 'Encyclopedie' in the period 1751–1772 together advocated scientific knowledge. This type of knowledge influenced thinking about the nature of humans and their ways of understanding the world and from this came an opening of the debate about what is knowledge and how humans can 'know' things.

Knowledge and evidence are inextricably linked – evidence provides support for the usefulness of certain types of knowledge and knowledge gives reason and value to different forms of evidence. Therefore, as with knowledge there are many different forms of evidence, each of which will be valued in different ways in different contexts. This chapter will consider the issues surrounding the nature of knowledge, the different forms of evidence and how it is possible to identify what it is that you need to know in order to ensure your practice is evidence-based.

The nature of knowledge

Knowledge can be defined as 'the facts or experiences known by a person or group of people; specific information about a subject' (*Collins Dictionary*, 1998). Knowledge is broadly categorized into two types – **propositional** and **non-propositional**. Propositional or codified knowledge is said to be public knowledge and is often given a formal status by its inclusion in educational programmes. Non-propositional knowledge is personal knowledge linked to experience and is described by Eraut (2000) as a 'cognitive resource' – a way of making sense of things – that someone will bring to any given situation to help them think and act. It is often linked to **tacit** knowledge. This is knowledge which is often difficult to put into words. For instance, you may know how to ride a bike and know how you learnt to do this, but may not be able to describe the critical aspects, such as how you manage to keep your balance.

In considering where knowledge comes from Kerlinger (1973) has identified three sources – **tenacity**, **authority** and **a priori**. Tenacity relates to knowledge that is believed simply because it has always held as the truth. Authority relates to knowledge which comes from a source or person viewed as being authoritative and therefore this must be true. A priori knowing relates to reasoning processes, where it is reasonable to consider something to be true. It is suggested that all three sources of knowledge are viewed as being objective in nature and not based on a person's subjective view of the world (see Box 2.1 for examples of these types of knowledge).

Box 2.1   Example of three sources of knowledge

An individual with a cold knows that taking cough mixture will soothe their cough. If asked how they know this they might answer:

- 'Because I know it does' – tenacity.
- 'Because my mother told me it does' – authority.
- 'Because it stands to reason that cough medicine will soothe a cough' – a priori.

Scientific knowledge

The term **science** comes from the Latin word *scietia* which means knowledge. Such knowledge has traditionally been seen as being based on observation, experiment and measurement (Mason and Whitehead, 2003). Scientific knowledge is usually generated either through **deductive** or **inductive reasoning** (Speziale and Carpenter, 2007). Deductive reasoning is said to move from the general to the particular, while inductive goes from the particular to the general. With deductive reasoning a nurse would start with a **hypothesis** which she would then seek to prove. A hypothesis is a simple statement that identifies a cause and effect relationship between two things – if I do X then

Y is likely to happen. For example, in relation to considering the use of wound dress-ings (the general issue) she might consider that one form of dressing (the particular) is more effective than another. The hypothesis might be that *wound dressing A will promote more rapid wound healing than dressing B*. In inductive reasoning, a nurse might start by considering somebody's experience of leg ulcers (a specific issue); she could then inter-view various people who have the condition, asking them about their experiences. Once a number of views have been collected it is possible to draw conclusions and a general theory of the experience could then be developed.

Deductive reasoning is often associated with **positivism**, the idea that reality is ordered, regular, can be studied objectively and quantified. A basic component of positivism is **empiricism**, where it is proposed that only that which can be observed can be called fact or truth. Originally such observation was intended to mean observation by the human senses – sight, touch, and so on. However, over time this has been expanded to include indirect observation through the use of specific tools designed to help a scientist observe and record phenomena. So whereas the study of personality could be viewed as impossible because you can't see it, the development of a personality inventory provides a tool that the scien-tist can use to study it empirically. The idea of 'cause and effect' is also important in empiricism – if I do this (cause) then this (effect) will happen – so, for exam-ple, if dressing X is used (cause) the wound will heal more quickly (effect). Empiricism is often described as reductionist, which relates to the breaking down of areas of interest into small parts rather than considering the whole.

Inductive reasoning is linked with **interpretivism**, an alternative to positivism based on the belief that humans are actively involved in constructing their understanding of the world. It is proposed that individuals constantly strive to understand what is happening in their environment and interpret action and interaction in an effort to make sense of their experiences. From this perspective, it is proposed that there are a range of views of the world and ways of under-standing, depending on the interpretation people give to their experiences. Rather than adopting reductionist approaches and identifying cause and effect, interpretivism is seen as considering the whole, exploring all the meanings and seeking a full as possible understanding of phenomena.

As can be seen from the above, philosophical positions are adopted about the nature of the world, what can be known and how to gather this knowledge. These philosophical positions are known as **paradigms**, a term created by Kuhn (1970). A paradigm is a set of logically connected ideas which guide the way in which research can be conducted – the methods used, the form of data collected, and how that data are analyzed. Two paradigms are generally accepted as being present in research – *qualitative* and *quantitative* – based on two different and sometimes competing ways of discovering the world. Qualitative research is concerned with exploring the meanings people attach to experiences and generating theories, whereas quantitative is focused on generating data to prove or disprove theories. The paradigms are reflected in the way data are collected – qualitative data tend to be in the form of words, what people say about their experiences; quantitative data are presented in the form of numbers providing a basis for statistical analysis. Examples of how research into the same general area might look are given in Table 2.1.

Quantitative methods include randomised control trials (RCTs) and experi-mental designs and also involve the statistical analysis of data. Qualitative enquiry

Table 2.1   *Examples of research questions*

An investigation of anxiety in patients	
What is the nature of anxiety in patients? What sorts of things provoke anxiety and what is the relationship between them?	Are patients who are supplied with information less anxious than those who are not?
This is a qualitative approach ... the question is a 'what IS this?' type. Suggests an inductive approach, moving from the specific to the general.	This requires a quantitative approach ... Suggests a cause and effect relationship and then tests it.

Table 2.2   *Differences between quantitative and qualitative research*

Quantitative	Qualitative
Scientific principles	Understanding/meaning of events
Moves from theory to data	Moves from data to theory
Identification of causal relationships between data	A close understanding of the research context
Collection of adequate amount of data	Collection of 'rich/deep' data
Application of controls to ensure validity	Seeks to address all aspects of the issues
Highly structured	Flexible structure allowing for changes in emphasis
Objectivity	Researcher as part of the process
Acceptance/rejection of hypothesis/laws	Generation of theory

includes phenomenology, ethnography, action research and grounded theory, and generally involves interviews and observation although some forms may incorporate aspects of statistical analysis. Table 2.2 provides a brief summary of the difference between qualitative and quantitative approaches. Issues related to the research approaches are discussed in further detail in Chapter 6 and 7.

Nursing knowledge

There is much debate as to what constitutes nursing knowledge. Knowledge plays a complex role in professions, often being seen as a defining trait. Schon (1987) suggested there is a hierarchy of knowledge in professions:

- basic science;
- applied science;
- technical skills of everyday practice.

He also suggested that professional status is dependent on this hierarchy, that the closer a professional knowledge base is to basic science the higher the status. Nursing has tried for many years to establish a defined scientific knowledge base. Huntington and Gilmour (2001) stated that nursing has traditionally focused on empirical approaches to knowledge generation and has used these to explain the nature of nursing practice. The development of this knowledge has been influenced by other disciplines such as medicine, psychology and sociology. Although for a number of years scientific knowledge has been accepted as superior to other forms, more recently this has been challenged and there is a growing belief that other forms of knowledge are essential to the practice of nursing.

Carper (1978) was one of the first people to provide a framework by which the patterns of knowing in nursing could be considered. She identified four types of nursing knowledge – *empirical, personal, aesthetic and ethical* – and suggested that no one form of knowledge was superior to the other, instead each was essential to the practice of nursing. Empirical knowledge is seen here as the theoretical and research-based knowledge which is generated through systematic investigation and observation. This may also be knowledge generated by other disciplines which can be seen as either a theory underpinning practice (such as anatomy and physiology) or a theory translated for a use in nursing in unique ways (as with applied sciences such as psychology). Chinn and Kramer (2004) added the development of nursing theory to the concept of empirical knowledge, particularly in relation to interpretive research approaches such as phenomenology.

Personal knowledge relates to an individual nurse's experience of the world generally and nursing specifically. It encompasses that person's beliefs, values, perceptions and level of self-awareness. In many ways it resembles reflective practice, as implicit within this is the ability to know yourself and how this influences your practice. The emotional aspects of nursing require nurses to consider how and why they respond to certain situations in certain ways to ensure the care they deliver is appropriate and compassionate. This type of knowledge is something that is seen as changing over time and having direct implications on the type and form of interactions that occur between nurses and the patients.

Aesthetic knowledge is described as that knowledge which underpins the 'art' of nursing. It can be seen as the bringing together of the manual, technical and intellectual skills aspects of nursing, particularly in nurse and patient interactions. This type of knowledge is often linked to expert practice and the ability to assist individuals in coping with health issues in a positive way. Finally ethical knowledge is seen as focusing on what is right, appropriate and moral: it relates to the judgements to be made in relation to nursing actions. It is also related to codes of conduct, procedural guidelines and the philosophical principles that underpin nursing.

ACTIVITY

Reflect on a recent clinical placement. Can you identify specific incidents where you used Carper's four types of knowledge?

Table 2.3 gives examples of some activities associated with the different types of knowledge identified by Carper.

Table 2.3 *Examples of activities associated with different types of knowledge*

Knowledge	Example
Empirical	Biological sciences knowledge to understand blood pressure readings
	Psychology theory in relation to phobias to understand a patient's fear of injections/needles
Personal	'Therapeutic use of self' in understanding a person's response when given 'bad news'
	Interpersonal relationships, therapeutic relationships
Ethical	Code of conduct
	Confidentiality
Aesthetic	Communicating with a patient in a caring and appropriate way before giving an injection
	Recognizing the individual needs of a person when helping them with personal hygiene

Intuition is one area that has been the subject of much debate, with what is termed **intuitive knowledge** being seen by many as an important aspect of nursing practice. Intuition can be defined as the 'instant understanding of knowledge without evidence of sensible thought' (Billay et al., 2007: 147) and is often considered to be a form of tacit knowledge. It is the moment when you 'know' that something is going to happen, or reach a conclusion, without being aware of thinking in a rational and logical way to arrive at that point. In considering the nature of intuition in professional practice, Benner (1984) suggested that a form of practice knowledge or 'expertise' exists which is part of expert practise. Here a nurse will draw on all her empirical and personal knowledge to reach a conclusion, without being aware of processing the information (see Box 2.2 for an example). Benner differentiated between practical and theoretical knowledge, suggesting that the former related to 'knowing how' and skills, and the latter to 'knowing that' which related to the generation of theory and scientific knowledge. However, she also suggested that in nursing, as expertise develops, a form of practice knowledge is apparent that 'sidesteps' the logical reasoning processes associated with science. Extending the knowing how of practice through practice experience can lead to knowledge that appears to be available to the person without the aid of an analytical process, but which nevertheless remains valid.

Box 2.2   Example of expert knowledge (Benner 1984: 32)

An extract from an interview from a nurse who worked in the psychiatric setting for 15 years:

When I say to a doctor 'this patient is psychotic', I don't always know how to legitimize that statement. But I am never wrong. Because I know psychosis from inside out. And I feel that, and I know it, and I trust it. I don't care if nothing else is happening, I still really know that. It's like the feeling another nurse described in the small group interview today, when she said about the patient 'she just isn't right.'

Finally socio-political knowledge (White, 1995) has more recently been included as a facet of nursing knowledge. Here political awareness, cultural diversity and public health agendas are seen as essential aspects of knowing, enabling nursing to see its practice in a broader arena.

What constitutes evidence?

The dictionary definition of evidence is 'grounds for belief or disbelief; data on which to base proof or establish truth or falsehood' (*Collins*, 1998). Upshur et al. (2001: 93) expanded this to 'an observation, fact or organized body of fact offered to support or justify inferences or beliefs in the demonstration of some proposition or matter at issue'. What exactly constitutes evidence in EBP is still hotly debated. Thomas (2004) suggested that evidence is information that is seen as relevant to how to provide care and beliefs about health and illness. Various hierarchies of evidence have been generated which clearly place quantitative findings from systematic reviews of RCTs at the top of the hierarchy, often qualitative research findings are not included within these hierarchies at all (see Box 2.3 for examples of a hierarchy). This preference for one form of evidence over another perhaps comes from the Cochrane Collaboration, which focused on the effectiveness of interventions for which RCTs are ideally suited and also on the dominance of the positivist paradigm in terms of research approaches.

Box 2.3   Examples of a hierarchy of evidence

1. Systematic reviews of RCTs.
2. Well designed RCTs.
3. Other types of experimental studies – pre-post test, cohort, time series.
4. Non-experimental studies.
5. Descriptive studies, expert committee reports.

However, there is a growing body of literature that hotly contests the placing of RCT methods at the top of the hierarchy. Petticrew and Roberts (2003) argued that RCTs are not always the most appropriate approach to certain issues. Different types of research question require different forms of study. Therefore the most appropriate form of evidence is that which relates to the question being asked – 'horses for courses', as they put it.

Nursing has long since recognized that its practice is based on multiple ways of knowing (Tarlier, 2004) and much of nursing's activities do not fit easily with an RCT approach. The advocating of one type of evidence as superior to another is not helpful in providing evidence on which to base practice in a profession as multifaceted and complex as nursing. Higgs and Jones (2000: 311) proposed that evidence in EBP is 'knowledge derived from a variety of sources that have been subjected to testing and found to be credible'. The Joanna Briggs Institute (JBI) supports the idea of there being a range of issues that need to be considered in health care, and that different forms of evidence are needed. They suggest that evidence generally falls into four areas:

1. Evidence of feasibility – whether something is practical/practicable physically, culturally or financially. In this situation one type of treatment might be the most effective, but financially unaffordable. For example, the cost of certain drugs means they are not used in some health-care systems. Types of evidence to support this would probably include economic and policy research.
2. Evidence of appropriateness – whether a particular intervention fits with the context in which it is to be given. For example, blood transfusion with certain religious groups might not be an appropriate form of treatment. Research considering ethical and philosophical issues would be of use here.
3. Meaningfulness – how interventions/activities are experienced by individuals. For example, patients' experiences of, or beliefs about, fertility treatment might influence how services are organized. Interpretive research in the form of phenomenology, ethnology or grounded theory would be of interest here.
4. Effectiveness – whether one treatment is better than another or the usual intervention. RCTs and cohort studies would be of use here.

Rycroft-Malone et al. (2004a) suggested there were four types of evidence on which nurses can base their practice:

- research;
- clinical experience;
- service user/carer perspectives;
- local context.

They went on to identify that the challenge is in knowing how to integrate these four types of evidence in a robust and patient-centred way.

Ensuring the robustness of evidence related to clinical experience requires the gathering and documenting of this experience in a systematic manner, allowing for individual and group reflection and cross-checking. Portfolios and clinical supervision are methods which can enhance the validity of this type of evidence and these are explored further in Chapter 10.

Incorporating sources of evidence from service users and carers into the delivery of care has had a long tradition within nursing and underpins the ethos of holistic care. This aspect is explored further in Chapter 3, however it has to be said that this source of evidence has its own inherent complexities and can be challenging. When research findings promote the view that a specific form of intervention is most appropriate (for example, the use of a particular medication in managing mental health problems) or is at odds with the service user experience (the medication has specific side effects that make the person unwilling to take it), the clinical expertise of the nurse involved will be essential in identifying the most appropriate course of action.

Institutional cultures, social and professional networks, evaluations such as 360° feedback, and local/national policies are some of the forms of evidence found in the local setting (Rycroft-Malone et al., 2004a). Other relevant local evidence will include audits and individual patient preferences and service evaluation.

There are also some 'ready-made' forms of evidence available, where best evidence has been collected and summarized for use by health-care professionals. Clinical Knowledge Summaries is an example of this type of resource. This is an on-line collection of concise summaries of available evidence, providing recommendations on how to manage commonly encountered clinical situations in primary care settings (www.cks.library.nhs.uk.)

A relatively new initiative in EBP is that of **care bundles**. Here elements of best practice evidence (usually between three and five items) are grouped together in relation to a particular condition, treatment and/or procedure. These elements are ones that are generally used in practice but not necessarily applied in the same way or combination to all appropriate patients. Care bundles 'tie' together these elements into a unit that can be delivered to every patient in the same way. Fulbrook and Mooney (2003) identified that combining these elements in this way can have a more positive impact on treatment outcomes than any one element alone. The idea is based on the holistic premise that 'the whole is greater than the sum' (2003: 250). Care bundles were originally developed in the USA at Johns Hopkins University in relation to critical care environments. It was found that using four interventions with patients on ventilators significantly reduced their length of stay and number of ventilator days. Care bundles have been developed in a number of areas and are now advocated by the Department of Health as a tool for high impact change.

Questions

Having identified what counts as good evidence, the next task is to find the evidence. This requires the formulating of a relevant question, often considered the backbone of EBP. Ideas in relation to questions about practice can come from a range of situations, reflection on practice issues, audit outcomes, and discussions between nurse, patients, and/or other health professionals. Often such questions are broad and unfocused, but if appropriate answers are to be found then there is a need to be specific as to what it is you want to know.

ACTIVITY: SCENARIO

You are currently working in a long-term care setting. Mary, a 66-year-old patient in your care, has fallen and fractured her femur. In discussion with the rest of the ward staff it is noted that there have been a number of patient falls over the year that have resulted in fractured femurs. Someone remembers reading about 'hip protectors' as a method of reducing injuries. You have been asked to look for some evidence to help make decisions on how to address the issue. Where would you start?

You might start here by going on line and Googling 'fractured femur', but you are likely to quickly discover that this either produces thousands of hits or nothing at all. You need to focus your search to ensure that you find the relevant information while at the same time not missing other vital pieces of information.

Sackett et al. (2000) identified that there are two forms of questions that practitioners might ask – **background** and **foreground**. Background questions are generally broad and will have two parts:

- the question's stem – who, what, where, when, how, why;
- the area of clinical interest.

A background question might look at something like *What is the best way of treating depression?* There is a need to ask a background question, particularly for students and those new to an area of practice, in order to gain the knowledge and expertise needed in relation to a specific area. The problem with background questions is their broadness which makes it difficult to find specific information, and searching for information is often done in a haphazard way – you can easily end up looking in the wrong place.

Foreground questions ask about specific issues and are looking for particular knowledge. A foreground question might be something like *Which is more effective in treating depression – cognitive behavioural therapy or medication?* It is essential that you formulate a foreground question containing all the key elements for consideration, before searching the literature in relation to a particular issue. The question will be central to ensuring that your search is not too broad, which in turn may result in you retrieving an overwhelming amount of literature, or too narrow, resulting in key items being missed. There are a number of formats that can be used to help to create a search question; the most commonly used is **PICO** (see Table 2.4).

Table 2.4   *Outline of PICO*

Population	Intervention	Comparison	Outcome

Include:
1. Disease/condition
   e.g. cancer/stroke.
 	
2. Population (e.g. age)
   and setting
   (e.g. community)
	Type of activity/
	procedure/treatment
	or action, e.g.
	use of a specific
	assessment tool
	
	Particular type of
	wound dressing
	
	Using a particular
	approach such as
	cognitive behavioural
	therapy
		Alternative activities
		or actions against
		which you compare
		your intervention:
		sometimes this might
		be usual treatment
			Results of a
			specified action
			
			All possible
			outcomes are
			explored

As you can see from Table 2.4:

P = population and could be something like *adult males with depression.*
I = intervention and could be something like *cognitive behavioural therapy.*
C = comparison and could be something like *antidepressant medication.*
O = outcome and could be something like *raised mood.*

The PICO question would then be:

In adult male service users diagnosed with depression is CBT more effective than antidepressants in treating depression?

In some instances the use of an extra letter such as T is added, which relates to the time frame over which the intervention would be observed, making PICOT. In the above question, for example, you could add *'over a period of 18 months'*. In other instances the letter S will be added, giving the acronym PICOS, with the S = Study type providing the opportunity to limit the type of the study you would want to include in your search of the literature. In this case you might only want to consider RCTs.

ACTIVITY

Consider the previous scenario about Mary, and apply the PICO principles. What question do you think would enable you to search for appropriate evidence?

It might look something like this:

In female adults over 65 years of age, is the use of hip projection more effective than normal precautions in reducing the incidence of fractured femurs following a fall?

A PICO framework tends to be most useful when asking 'effectiveness' questions and reflects the quantitative approach to research. However, it is less helpful for considering qualitative aspects of care such as patient experiences. The JBI offers an alternative formation – PICo:

Participants
phenomena of **Interest**
Context

If in relation to the above scenario you were actually interested in patients' experiences of wearing hip protectors, in this instance the question might be:

In female adults over 65 yrs of age (P), what is their experience of wearing hip protectors (I) in a hospital setting (Co)?

Formulating questions in this way will enable you to focus on what is the real question that needs to be addressed and will help you to move on to the next stage of the process – searching for the evidence. The question will provide you with the key terms to be used in the search.

EBP ACTIVITY

Think about a recent clinical experience and identify a patient whose care you were closely involved with. Focusing on one clinical intervention you undertook in relation to this person (giving an injection, attending to hygiene needs, an involvement in recreational activities) write a reflective account identifying:

1. What knowledge you were using during the intervention/activity, considering what areas of knowledge you felt most comfortable with and those that you need to develop further.
2. What evidence you used to direct how you organized your intervention/activity.
3. The questions you would ask if you wanted to find further evidence to support your practice in this area.

SUMMARY

- Knowledge is broadly categorized into two types – propositional (formal) and non-propositional (personal) – and comes from three sources: tenacity, authority and a priori.
- Science is a body of knowledge organized in a systematic way and based on observation, experiment and measurement.
- Evidence is information or data which supports or refutes beliefs in relation to a particular area of interest.
- Evidence on which to base nursing practice is best drawn from a variety of credible sources, thereby reflecting the multifaceted and complex needs of nursing. There are four types of evidence on which nurses can base their practice – research, clinical experience, service user/carer perspectives and local context.
- There are also some 'ready-made' forms of evidence available where best evidence has been collected and summarized, such as clinical guidelines and summaries.
- Appropriate and focused questions forms the backbone of EBP. The PICO format is suggested as helpful in the development of questions related to effectiveness, while PICo is suitable for those related to feasibility, meaning and appropriateness.

Further reading

Carper, B. (1978) 'Fundamental patterns of knowing in nursing', *Advances in Nursing Science*, 1: 13–23. Useful for a full exploration of the nature of nursing knowledge.

Fulbrook, P. and Mooney, S. (2003) 'Care bundles in critical care: A practice approach to evidence based practice', *Nursing in Critical Care*, 8 (6): 249–55. Gives a step-by-step account of care bundles.

Miller, S.A. and Forrest, J.J. (2001) 'Enhancing your practice decision making: PICO, good questions', *Journal of Evidence-Based Dental Practice*, 1: 136–41. Helpful for further exploration of using PICO in question formation.

E-resources

Critical Appraisal Skills Programme: provides a range of resources to help with developing
   the skills associated with EBP. Also provides a range of critical appraisal tools.
www.phru.nhs.uk/Pages/PHD/CASP.htm

Netting the evidence: aimed at promoting evidence-based health care and providing
   resources to support evidence-based activities.
http://www.shef.ac.uk/scharr/ir/netting/

3

Patients' Perspectives and Clinical Judgement

Introduction

The NHS Plan (DoH 2001) set out a ten-year programme for improving health-care services in Britain. It identified three phases to this improvement, putting in place the structures to ensure such services were delivered appropriately; making the service more responsive to the needs of modern society; and promoting safe and clinically effective care which would enhance patient experience. Central to all these phases is the involvement of service users in the decisions made about their care and the development of sound clinical decision-making skills in nurses. As seen in Chapter 1 these aspects are also central to EBP and are key issues when considering the use of evidence in your daily practice.

Portney (2004) has suggested that EBP should more correctly be called evidence-based decision making, as it requires practitioners to draw on a range of information and make a decision as to what is actually required. However, decision making is not a straightforward activity and can be very complex. EBP does not happen in a vacuum; there is a need to consider evidence in light of:

- the specific setting in which it is to be applied;
- individual client(s) needs, values, beliefs and choices;
- your development in clinical decision-making skills and knowledge;
- the resources available to facilitate the use of specific forms of evidence in your practice.

Therefore these concepts will be explored and the relationship between scientific knowledge and practice experience debated.

Patients' perspectives

There is a tension between EBP as a scientific approach to care – based on sound evidence – and the underlying health philosophy of being patient-centred, requiring nursing in particular to respond holistically to the individual needs of patients. However, Sidani (2006) suggested the two approaches are complementary as both aim at ensuring that care is acceptable to the patient and delivered in the most effective way. The concept of patient involvement requires health professionals to recognize the active role of patients in ensuring health care is safe, effective and meets their needs. Service users expect to be involved in decisions related to their health treatment options and care 'as equals with different expertise' (Command Paper, 2001).

As identified above, service user involvement is central to government policy. In 2003 the Department of Health document, 'Building on the Best: Choice, Responsiveness and Equity in the NHS', reported on a consultation of over 110,000 people and identified that people want to be involved in the decisions made about their health and health care. The type of experience patients wanted from the NHS was defined as:

- getting good treatment in a comfortable, caring and safe environment, delivered in a calm and reassuring way;
- having information to make choices, to feel confident and to feel in control;
- being talked to and listened to as an equal and treated with honesty, respect and dignity.

This definition appears to incorporate the essential elements of patient-centred care (see Box 3.1). Amongst the various commitments made by the government in this document is a pledge to 'ensure people have the right information, at the right time, with the support they need to use it so that this becomes central to how we care for people' (DoH, 2003: 9). Yet there is strong evidence to suggest that patients continue to have little input into the decisions made about their treatment and care (see, for example, Pollock et al., 2004).

Box 3.1   Characteristics of patient-centred care

- Recognizing the patient as a unique individual with specific
  - beliefs/values;
  - needs;
  - preferences;
  - experience;
  - concerns.

- Responding flexibly to the patient in the provision of care, ensuring it reflects his/her individual

    - needs;
    - preference;
    - concerns.

Table 3.1   *Models of user involvement*

Model	Description
Consumerist	<ul><li>Emerged in the late 1980s/early 1990s.</li><li>Service users seen as customers and/or consumers of the health services.</li><li>Emphasized increased choice.</li></ul>
Democratic	<ul><li>Appeared in mid-1990s.</li><li>Sought to equal the balance of power between professionals and patients, by empowering service users.</li><li>Advocated the involvement of service users in decision-making.</li></ul>
Stakeholder	<ul><li>Grew out of the democratic approach in the late 1990s.</li><li>Emphasizes a partnership between all stakeholders – patients, professionals, government – to ensure all have equal influence on the development of services and delivery of care.</li></ul>

Traditionally the model of care in a health setting is what is termed 'paternalistic', where it is expected that patients will comply with the 'orders' of health professionals. However, shared decision-making is seen to provide better health outcomes, better adherence to treatment regimes and higher levels of patient satisfaction (Doherty and Doherty, 2005). Therefore it would seem both clinically and cost effective to promote some form of partnership working between service users and health professionals. Three models of service user involvement have been proposed (see Table 3.1), but the basic foundation of all three is to ensure that patients are included at various levels of the decision-making processes (Barker and Rush, 2009).

Patients' preferences and experiences can be gained in two ways – from individual patients or via collations of multiple sources. There are a number of possible ways in which to gather a general understanding of collated patients' preferences (see Box 3.2). These can give a general insight into how patients view certain aspects of care; what might impact on the uptake of treatment and the continuation of treatment regimes; and the factors that lead to dissatisfaction. This information can also be useful when discussing options with individual patients as it can provide a background for discussion and exploring specific issues that may be of concern to individuals. It can also provide a source of information to include in your decision-making processes, by identifying possible issues you may need to take into consideration which individual patients have not identified.

Box 3.2   Collated patients' perspectives

- Research studies considering patient opinions.
- Local service user organizations (e.g., Help the Aged in the case of older people, MIND for mental health topics).
- National bodies (e.g., Long Term Conditions Alliance, Patients Association, Expert Patient Programme, Sainsbury Centre for Mental Health).
- Own institution's audits and service evaluation reports.

ACTIVITY

Select a topic of interest related to the delivery of care in your area of practice. Choose and locate two sources of information as identified in Box 3.2 and point out potential patients' perspectives in relation to that topic area.

Accessing individual preferences from patients in your care and attempting to integrate patient preferences in to clinical decision-making is central to EBP. Sidani (2006) identified this as a three-step process:

1. Identifying evidence on which to base care, accounting for alternative approaches to meet patient needs and preparing easy to understand descriptions of that evidence.
2. Informing patients of the possible options and identifying preferences.
3. Integrating patient preferences into the delivery of care.

As Step 1 indicates, it is essential that you have full information regarding the proposed intervention(s) so you can ensure the patient has a complete understanding of the issues. Preparing a written description is often helpful as it can allow the patient to consider the information in a format that they can return to and take in at their own pace. (Appendix 2 provides a possible template for providing this information.)

ACTIVITY

Identify an aspect of care relevant to your own area. Prepare a description of that aspect of care using the template provided in Appendix 2.

Alternatively, standardized patient decision tools are available to help facilitate patients' decision-making. These tools are usually generated following clinical research and studies of patients' information needs and can guide patients through the decision-making process in a step-by-step way (O' Connor et al., 2004). It is intended that these will be used when there is more than one possible option available in relation to a particular health issue. Each aid presents the various risks and benefits of each option in a clear and simple way, enabling patients to make an informed choice based on their own preferences and values.

Decision aids can come in many forms – leaflets, interactive software, workbooks – and are intended to be used by health professionals to inform their discussions rather than replace them. It is believed that such decision aids do three things: provide an overview of the facts relating to the intervention option; help people to clarify their preferences and values; and provide a means of communicating these to health professionals. The Cochrane Review Team of Patient Decision Aids have created and reviewed decision aids, and a register of these can be found on the collaboration site (www.ohri.ca/decisionaids).

ACTIVITY

Visit the Decision Aids website and identify a tool relevant to your area of practice. Consider whether this tool would be useful in helping you to gain an overview of a patient's preferences and how you might implement it.

Gaining a patient's perspective requires giving your full attention to that individual's 'narrative' – their story – and enabling them to freely express their beliefs, values and concerns in a non-judgemental and supportive way. This requires you to have good communication and interpersonal skills and the ability to build a trusting relationship with the patient. It is not in the remit of this chapter to consider these issues in any depth. However, Kitson (2002) has suggested there are basic skills underpinning this activity:

- knowing what questions to ask;
- using active listening skills;
- having an awareness of the principles underpinning patient-centred care (PCC);
- putting the principles of PCC into practice;
- being open to new ideas and alternative ways of thinking;
- making explicit links between different sources of knowledge, evidence and decision-making processes.

ACTIVITY

Choose one of the Kitson's basic (2002) skills identified above. Undertake a SWOT analysis - see the template in Appendix 1 - in relation to your skills in this area. Then develop an action plan identifying how you will develop this aspect in order to enhance your EBP activities.

Patients' participation in decision-making is not without its problems. It has been identified that not all patients want to be involved in such decision-making processes. Whilst it is essential that they are provided with the appropriate information and informed consent is obtained before any care is delivered, it must be remembered that patients also have the right to choose what level of involvement they wish to have (Doherty and Doherty, 2005). Alternatively, problems may be encountered if a patient's preference runs counter to what is thought to be the most effective or feasible treatment or they choose an option that it is thought will be detrimental to their well-being.

What is clinical judgement?

Clinical judgement is an essential skill for all health professionals and one that separates them from undertaking a purely technical role. Various terms are used in relation to this activity (clinical reasoning, diagnostic reasoning) but all are related to the ability to consider the various issues at hand, make a judgement in relation to the impact of the various elements, and come up with a decision in terms of what is the appropriate action to take.

Melnyk and Fineout-Overholt (2005) have suggested it is useful to think of EBP as requiring you to be involved in two essential activities – critically appraising evidence (discussed in Chapter 5) and using clinical judgement to consider how applicable the evidence is to your own area of practice. There is a need to consider how the evidence relates to your context of practice – is it transferable, and are there identifiable risks and/or benefits to using the evidence in your area of practice? There needs to be a weighing up of options with an acceptance that decisions made may vary from patient to patient in the same situations. For example, research evidence may suggest a certain course of action is appropriate for women aged between 50 and 60 with leg ulcers. However, in reality one woman may be reluctant to receive treatment, and may have perfectly valid reasons for this concern, whilst another could be perfectly happy to accept the intervention.

ACTIVITY

Reflect on a recent practice experience where some patients appeared more accepting of a particular aspect of care than others. What factors may have impacted on those patients' willingness to accept care?

Tanner (2006: 204) defined clinical judgement as 'an interpretation or conclusion about a patient's needs … and/or the decision to take action', and suggested that there are various factors that can impact on this process:

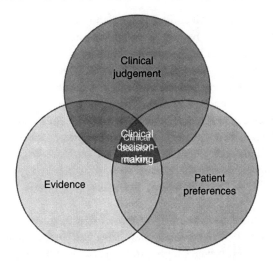

Figure 3.1   *Components of clinical decision-making*

- nurses' experiences and perspectives/values – these can have a greater impact on clinical judgement than scientific evidence;
- a knowledge of the patient and their preferences;
- the context and culture of the care environment.

Benner et al. (1996: 2) suggested that clinical judgement related to 'the ways in which nurses come to understand the problems, issues, or concerns of clients/patients, to attend to salient information and to respond in concerned and involved ways'. In this way decision-making is seen as an interaction between three things – the patient's preferences, the evidence available on which to base practice and the clinical judgement of the nurse involved based on their personal experience and knowledge. These three components can then come together to produce a clinical decision as to what action should be taken (see Figure 3.1).

A conceptual model to explain the factors involved in making a clinical decision has been identified by Tanner (2006). She proposed a four-stage process involving noticing, interpreting, responding and reflecting. Lasater (2006) also identified that each of these stages has specific components.

- noticing – observing, noticing change and collecting information;
- interpreting – making sense of the information and prioritizing;
- responding – planning an intervention, using clear communication and appropriate skills;
- reflecting – evaluating the incident and looking for ways to improve performance.

Harbison (2006) suggested that practitioners consider evidence in terms of its relevance and weight, however this is an individual assessment so what might be considered relevant and given great weight by one clinician may not be considered in the same way by another. All clinical judgements will have ethical considerations, with the health professional having to weigh up the potential benefits and risks involved in any decision made. Frequently there are a number of options available, each of which carries their own risks and benefits. This also adds another dimension to the decision-making process and often it is the patient's preferences that will indicate which is the best choice. Therefore reflection is central to clinical judgement as it requires health professionals to consider and make links between the evidence, their own knowledge, skills and experience and that of other team members, as well as patient preferences, beliefs and values. However, for this to be effective in aiding clinical judgement it must be undertaken in a clear and structured way rather than simply 'thinking about' the issues. (Reflection is explored further in Chapter 10.)

In making a clinical decision, it is proposed that a nurse's judgement will be aided if the most up-to-date evidence is available and the needs of the service user are clearly identified. However, simply providing nurses with appropriate evidence will not in itself enhance the decision-making processes. Thompson (2003) put forward the notion of 'clinical uncertainty' in relation to decision-making – the idea that the practice of nursing takes place in the face of ever-changing demands. A patient's needs and status will change over time, thus resulting in complex and often competing demands.

If decision-making is to be effective then as a health professional you need to be aware of such changes and factor them into any decisions you must make. Therefore it is necessary to consider the implications of a decision over time, what Melnyk and Fineout-Overholt (2005) describe as 'clinical forethought'. This consists of four components – future think, forethought about specific populations, the anticipation of risks and the unexpected (see Table 3.2 for an overview). Issues that may have an impact on, and implications for, care delivery should be identified and considered.

ACTIVITY

Imagine you are about to administer a new form of medication to a patient for the first time. What 'clinical forethought' issues can you identify?

The form of uncertainties nurses face can be seen in the types of clinical questions that Thompson et al. (2002) identify nurses ask in clinical decision-making (see Table 3.3). Clinical judgement is used in managing these uncertainties and arriving at a decision as to how to proceed – many see this as the 'art' of nursing – and is central to clinical expertise.

As identified above, knowledge and experience have the greatest impact on these decision-making activities, moulding how a nurse interprets a situation and deals with the uncertainties. The greater the knowledge/experience, the larger the number of perspectives and possibilities the nurse is likely to identify. As Benner

Table 3.2   *Clinical forethought*

Type	Description
Future think	• Considering the immediate future and anticipating issues that might arise. • Identifying the immediate resources needed. • Considering future responses. • Evaluating judgement and making adjustments as necessary.
Specific patients	• Considering general trends in patient experiences and responses to intervention. • Identifying the local resources available to deal with potential issues.
Risks	• Anticipating particular issues that may impact on a specific individual – such as anxiety, distress, etc.
The unexpected	• Expecting the unexpected. • Anticipating the need to respond to new situations and resources – your own and organizational – that will be needed if difficulties arise.

Table 3.3   *Types of decision-making question (Thompson et al., 2002)*

Type	Example

Effectiveness
  – targeting
  – timing
	Is this intervention better than that one?
	Who would benefit from this intervention?
	When is it best to implement this intervention?

Communication	What is the best way to give certain information?
Service Delivery	What is the best way to manage, organize, and deliver care?
Experiential	What is the patient's experience of this care/process/intervention?

(1984) has already pointed out, the 'expert' nurse draws on knowledge in an intuitive way and reaches conclusions without being able to verbalize the process by which those decisions were reached (see Chapter 2 in relation to tacit knowledge). However, Fitzpatrick (2007) suggested that an expert nurse, in relation to EBP, needs to be able to make clear and reasoned links between theory and practice and to have the ability to integrate patient perspectives into this 'mix'.

Nursing expertise is defined by Titchen and Higgs (2001: 274) as the 'professional artistry and practice wisdom inherent in professional practice'. Clinical expertise is viewed by Manley et al. (2005) as having a number of components (see Box 3.3). The development of these aspects of clinical expertise is said to be linked to 'enabling factors' – the ability to reflect; to organize practice giving consideration to overarching influences; to work autonomously; to develop good interpersonal relationships; and to promote respect.

Box 3.3   Nursing expertise

1. Holistic practice knowledge – integrating various forms of knowledge (academic and experiential) into the delivery of care.
2. Knowing the patient – respecting the patient's views/perspectives, encouraging patient decision-making and promoting independence.
3. Moral agency promoting respect, dignity and self-efficacy in others whilst maintaining own professional integrity.
4. Saliency – observing and picking up on cues from patients, recognizing the needs of patients and others.
5. Skilled know-how – problem-solving, responding to the changing environment of care and adapting to needs as appropriate.
6. Change catalyst – promoting appropriate change.
7. Risk taker – weighing the risks and taking appropriate decisions to achieve best patient outcomes.

The reasoning processes used in clinical judgement tend to be described as involving either analytical or intuitive activities. The former involves breaking down a problem into its constituent parts, considering these, and then weighing up the alternative approaches available for solving that problem. Intuitive processes can be seen as drawing on inherent knowledge, skills and experiences to find the answer to a problem. These two options are often viewed as the opposite ends of a continuum, however it is rare that any decision is purely based on rational processes or is made completely on intuition. The idea of a 'cognitive continuum' is possibly more helpful in understanding the processes involved. It is also suggested that different approaches are used in different situations depending on the complexity, ambiguity and presentation of the issue. The more complex, familiar or urgent an issue is, the more likely you are to rely on your intuition. Any combination of these three elements will result in the use of differing levels of analysis and/or intuition.

ACTIVITY

Consider the last clinical decision you made. How did you arrive at that decision? Were you aware of analyzing the various aspects of the issue or was this reached more intuitively?

EBP calls for a more analytical approach to making clinical decisions, and it is anticipated there will be a conscious weighing up of the options and considerations of the various issues involved. The McMaster's EBM group cautions against the use of clinical experience and intuition in the absence of evidence based on systematic observation in making clinical judgements (Eraut, 2000). However, you should not underestimate how much interpretation may be needed in deciding how evidence should be used – EBP cannot always provide concrete evidence on which to base practice. A possible model for this process is given in Figure 3.2.

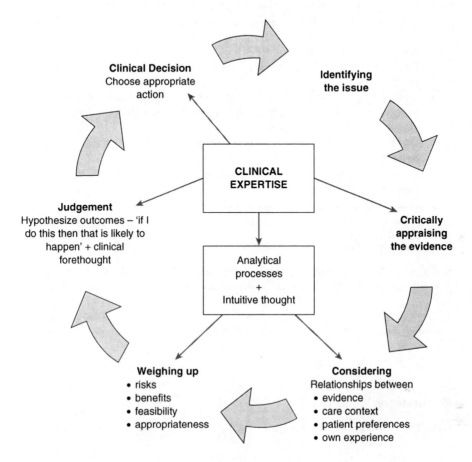

Figure 3.2   *Model for clinical decision-making*

EBP ACTIVITY

For a novice nurse there are three issues which may impact on their ability to successfully adopt evidence-based practices (Ferguson and Day, 2007):

1. Initial lack of practice-based knowledge.
2. Difficulty in identifying a patients' preferences and values.
3. Lack of confidence in their own clinical judgement and decision-making processes.

Complete a SWOT analysis of these three areas to enable you to identify your future learning needs.

SUMMARY

- Involving service users in decisions and using sound clinical decision-making are central to EBP. Patient involvement ensures health care is safe, effective and meets their needs – improving health outcomes, adherence to treatment and patient satisfaction.
- Communication and interpersonal skills are essential in obtaining patient preferences.
- Clinical judgement is seen as the 'art' of nursing and central to clinical expertise, and this involves the weighing up of options and reaching a decision as to appropriate action.
- There is a need to consider the impact of decisions for the future of the patient and their care delivery.
- Both analytical processes and intuitive thinking are central to clinical judgement.

Further reading

Kitson, A. (2002) 'Recognising relationships: Reflections on evidence-based practice', *Nursing Inquiry*, 9(3): 179–86. Offers an insight into the processes involved in making a clinical judgement.

Tanner, C.A. (2006) 'Thinking like a nurse: A research-based model of clinical judgement in nursing', *Journal of Nurse Education*, 45(6): 204–11. Gives an overview of decision-making processes.

E-resources

Long Term Condition Alliance: established in 1989, this provides a 'voice' for patients with long term conditions.
www.ltca.org.uk

Sainsbury Centre for Mental Health: aims to improve the quality of life for those experiencing mental health problems.
www.scnh.org.uk

Cochrane Collaboration of Patient Decision Aids (Ottawa Health Research Institute): provides a collection of patient decision aids.
www.ohri.ca/decisionaid

Finding the Evidence

Introduction

Searching for evidence can be both bewildering and complex. However, it is an important skill to develop and as Greenhalgh (2006) has already pointed out you may be rigorous in critically appraising the evidence but if you are considering the wrong paper then this is a waste of your time and effort. Most forms of evidence are now available electronically, so an important part of finding the evidence is being able to navigate your way through the various electronic systems involved. This chapter will introduce you to some of the key aspects related to finding the right evidence.

Where is the evidence?

Evidence is often thought of as being published materials only but it can take many forms. The value and credibility of each type have to be considered when trying to establish if it is going to be useful to you. Books are often the first point of access for many people and remain a useful source of background information. However, these do not always provide the most up-to-date evidence. Journals can supply a range of articles, from research papers to discussion pieces. Research studies, as we have already seen, are generally viewed as being important forms of evidence. Discussion and commentary papers can also be equally important when considering concepts and theories that are central to a profession's knowledge base or where little is known about a topic. In addition government and policy documents can prove a valuable source of information.

Another important source of evidence is what is known as **grey literature**. This is literature which has not been formally published, but nevertheless may include helpful information. Usually grey literature is said to include:

- theses and/or dissertations – projects undertaken as part of a course of study for various levels of degree (Masters and doctorates);
- conference proceedings which can provide information not available in print;
- in-house publications – leaflets, newsletters, pamphlets.

What resources are available to help with EBP

With the explosion of information and knowledge available on which to base practice, busy practitioners can find themselves overwhelmed and almost drowning in a sea of evidence. Hayes (2008) has put forward four resources available to help practitioners make decisions about integrating evidence into practice:

1. Systems.
2. Synopses.
3. Syntheses.
4. Studies.

He proposed that these are arranged in a hierarchical order with systems providing the highest and most useful form of information on which to base EBP. Systems are described as electronic records which can integrate and summarize all appropriate evidence related to a particular clinical issue such as clinical evidence (www.clinicalevidence.com). Synopses are summaries of individual studies, providing sufficient detail to make decisions as to whether something is relevant to your practice area and could be incorporated into clinical actions. These can be seen in the form of abstracts that appear in journals such as *Evidence-Based Nursing*. Syntheses, in the form of systematic reviews, which provide rigorous reviews of evidence relating to specific areas of interest, are also advocated as good sources of information. Finally, original studies investigating specific issues are the building blocks of all the other resources and often the starting point for EBP. However, you do need to have the skills and tools to enable you to find and use these resources.

Searching

Searching for evidence is a skill that takes time and practise to develop and it is important that you get all the help you can. Many of the tools discussed below will have tutorials that talk you through the steps you need to take to make best use of the resources. It is well worth spending some time working through these. I would also advise that you make friends with your local librarian, who can help you develop the skills you need. Also book a training session with the them, your personal tutor or the information technologist for your School or Health

Organization to work through the basics of navigating the electronic systems. It will be time well spent and save you a great deal of time and frustration later when you are searching for evidence to support your practice.

The first step in searching for evidence is deciding what it is you want to find, and as discussed in Chapter 2 you need to decide what your focus is and then identify a question using the PICO format. The terms you identify in PICO will help you narrow down what you are actually looking for and can then form the basis of the terms you will use to search for appropriate evidence. In searching there is a need to consider:

- synonyms – words that share the same meaning (e.g., cancer and neoplasm);
- acronyms – where phrases have been shortened to a set of letters (e.g., COPD – chronic obstructive pulmonary disease);
- alternative spellings (e.g., oedema and edema);
- alternative terms (e.g., learning disabilities and learning disorders).

ACTIVITY

Identify an area you would like to know more about and generate a PICO question. Look at the words or phrases you have identified and identify what other words may be associated with them.

You may come up with a long list or just a few phrases. Whichever is the case, these are what are known as your free text words/phrases. These are the words/phrases you can use to search for the evidence you need.

Manual searching

Your local library will have a range of resources that you can use to find the information you need. Most libraries will have an electronic database of the books, journals and other resources available to its members. Using the words you have generated should help you to locate the information you want. Don't underestimate the resources that libraries have available to them, the most valuable being the librarians themselves. Librarians, again, are a key resource in finding the information you need.

Electronic searching

Today most people search electronic databases to ensure that they have the most up-to-date information and to increase their awareness of what is actually available on a given topic. Whilst libraries are often the first port of call, the physical resources within them are limited and there is often a need to look more widely.

Search engines

Search engines are designed to search for information on the World Wide Web. Google is the most popular and well known search engine and can be a useful tool. However, it is not sufficiently focused to meet all your needs when looking for evidence on which to base your practice, and at the time of writing when I typed in the term 'learning disability' this produced 6,970,000 results. It is essential that you do not rely on general search engines such as Google and that you instead familiarize yourself with and use those that are specifically aimed at the health-care professions. See Box 4.1 for examples of commonly used search engines.

Box 4.1   Commonly used search engines

- Google and Google Scholar – provide access to electronic journal and text books
- Knowledge Finder – www.kfinder.com/newweb/
- Turning research into practice – a search engine for EBM (www.tripdatabase.com/)
- SUMSearch – searches various databases including MEDLINE, the National Guideline Clearing House, and DARE (http://sumsearch.uthscsa.edu/)

ACTIVITY

Choose and locate one of the search engines identified in Box 4.1 (not Google). Type in the 'search box' one of the text words generated in the earlier activity. How many 'hits' are identified? Consider whether the results are sufficiently focused to meet your needs in searching for evidence.

Gateway sites

A **gateway site** will provide access to resources, databases and publications associated with a specific topic area. Some of these are free while others will require a password. There are a growing number that are specific to the health-care professions. Box 4.2 outlines some of the most commonly used.

ACTIVITY

Repeat the above activity using one of the gateway sites identified in Box 4.2. Compare the results and consider the differences between the two sets of results.

Box 4.2   Gateway sites

- Intute for Health and Life Sciences – a free online service providing links to key education and research resources (note that this has replaced NMAP, the nursing, midwifery and allied health professions site). Available at www.intute.ac.uk/healthand lifesciences/
- National Library for Health (NLH) – an NHS funded service which provides access to a range of resources. Available at www.nlh.nhs.uk
- NHS Direct – another NHS site which provides various resources relevant to EBP. Available at www.nhsdirect.nhs.uk
- Social Sciences Information – Gateway (SOSIG) provides information related to the social sciences. Available at www.sosig.ac.uk

Databases

Databases are a central point where details relating to certain types of information are gathered together. The ones that are of interest here are those related to the health-care professions, and the most well known ones used are listed in Box 4.3 below. Those most commonly used by nurses are CINAHL and MEDLINE. Again, some of these are available for free but many will require a form of subscription. Your university or health organization will have a subscription to those it feels are of most use to learners and staff.

Box 4.3   Commonly used bibliographic databases

- CINAHL (Cumulative Index for Nursing and Allied Health Literature) – literature relating to nursing and allied health professions from over 2928 journals, dating back to 1982. In looking for evidence this is a key source of information and often the place most nurses start.
- MEDLINE – primary source for biomedical data from 1966 to the present. Compiled by the US National Libraries of Medicine.
- AMED – allied and complimentary database.
- EMBASE (Excerpta Medica Online) – similar to MEDLINE but having a focus on drugs and pharmacology.
- PsycINFO – has a database of publications which reaches back to the late nineteenth century related to psychology and allied fields such as mental health nursing and psychiatry.
- RCN (Royal College of Nursing) – has its own database accessible to members only.
- UKOP – UK official publication database and a useful site for grey literature.
- SIGLE – systems for information on grey literature.

(Continued)

(Continued)

- Cochrane Library – regularly updated systematic reviews.
- JBI – the Joanna Briggs Institute.
- DARE (database for abstracts of Reviews of Effect) – contains over 5000 appraisals of systematic reviews not found in the Cochrane database.
- SCOPUS – contains title, abstract and key words from numerous journals plus patents.
- NCG (National Guideline Clearance House) – indexes summaries of guidelines and links to full text versions.
- Dissertation Abstracts – a guide to US dissertations since 1861 and British dissertations for 50 universities since 1988.

Usually the information related to the content of the databases will be organized in a particular way. Bibliographic databases usually store publication information in the form of the title, author, book/journal title, year, journal volume, issue and page numbers. The full texts of articles are not usually available on these databases. However, once again your own education and/or health organization will have certain databases networked onto their computer system with links to access certain journals and information sources electronically. It is important that you are aware of what resources are available to you when searching for evidence.

Finding the literature you want

In searching electronically the words you have generated in relation to your PICO question are used to form what is known as a **search filter**. A search filter is the information you put into the database to find the sources of evidence you want. These can be simple or complex – you will see in Chapter 8 that extensive filters are used in systematic reviews. Some databases have filters built into them, while in others you will have to provide these yourself.

All databases use standard words to describe the content of articles, with the most well known being the medical subject headings commonly known as **MeSH terms**. Each database will have its own thesaurus or index structure – CINAHL, for example has 12714 subject headings which it states reflect the language used by health professionals. If you type a word or phrase into a database it will usually offer you alternative terms: these are the subject headings. When searching you can decide whether to go with your own phrase or to use the subject headings provided. You can also search for exact phrases through the use of quotation marks – " ". If for instance you want to retrieve information in relation to essential skills clusters, place this in the search box as "essential skills cluster", so only those publications containing the exact phrase will be retrieved.

ACTIVITY

Type the text words you identified earlier into a database of your choice. What alternative terms are offered? Consider whether these more closely describe you area of interest.

An alternative method of identifying subject headings, known as **Citation Pearl Growing,** is offered by Stott (1999). In this scenario you locate an article related to your area of interest that you already know about (the pearl) and look at the subject headings on the retrieved record – these are usually found by 'clicking' on the full/complete reference link. Those that appear relevant are used to locate similar articles, and the subject headings within them are then considered and added to the search strategy. If you don't have a 'pearl' to start with you can simply use your text words and then review the subject headings of the article records that are retrieved.

In choosing a subject heading you may be offered two further options – to focus or explode the heading. If you choose to focus the heading a series of subheadings will be given and you can restrict the search to certain areas. The articles that have the subheading(s) as their main focus are then retrieved. See Box 4.4 for an example of the focus terms generated for the subject heading 'learning disabilities'.

Box 4.4   Focus terms associated with the search words 'learning disabilities' on MEDLINE database (2008)

Blood	Metabolism
Chemically Induced	Microbiology
Classification	Mortality
Complications	Nursing
Diagnosis	Parasitology
Diet Therapy	Pathology
Drug Therapy	Physiopathology
Economics	Prevention & Control
Enzymology	Psychology
Epidemiology	Radiography
Ethnology	Radionuclide Imaging
Etiology	Rehabilitation
Genetics	Therapy
History	Urine
Immunology	

If you choose the 'explode' option it will provide a series of headings associated with the selected term which you can also include in your search. For instance the CINAHL thesaurus tree in relation to 'leg ulcer' is:

        Skin and connective tissue disease
          Skin disease
         Skin ulcer
           Fungating wound
            Leg ulcer
             Foot ulcer
              Venous ulcer
               Pressure ulcer
                Pyoderma gangrenosum

If you explode the search, all items – including the term 'leg ulcer' – and those listed below it will be retrieved.

Boolean terms

These are the words '*and*', '*or*' and '*not*', which are used to combine search terms. So for example if you are interested in literature in relation to Alzheimer's disease, you may consider using the terms 'Alzheimer's' and 'Dementia'. A search of MED-LINE using Boolean terms generated the following results:

- Dementia *and* Alzheimer's – 8571 articles containing both words.
- Dementia *or* Alzheimer's – 54,974 articles containing either of the terms.
- Dementia *not* Alzheimer's – 22,857 articles containing dementia and not Alzheimer's.

Clearly if you want articles related to dementia and Alzheimer's then using 'and' is the best option. However, if you are interested in dementia generally but not in Alzheimer's specifically, then 'not' might be the most appropriate term to use.

Truncation

Truncation allows you to search for words that may appear in various forms, without having to include them all in the search. It entails the use of truncation marks (often $ or ★) after a stem word. Rather than looking for 'fall', 'falls', 'falling', you could simply put 'fall★' or 'fall$'. However, the downside here is that this type of searching generates lots of results as any passing reference to a word is retrieved. For example, when I searched CINAHL for 'dementia' and 'fall★', 558 records of various publications were returned, but when I looked at the first ten results two articles focusing on dementia had been retrieved that were entirely irrelevant: one because of the author's name – Fallon – and another because the abstract included the term 'fall into line'.

Wildcards

Where words may have various spellings – such as paediatric and pediatric – a symbol (often ?) can be placed in the word at the point where the variation may occur. In this case 'p?ediatric' would be the case. Words with that spelling will be then searched for and retrieved.

Limiting

Most databases will allow you to limit your search in certain ways once your free text and/or subject headings have been accepted. You can limit your search in terms of publication dates – choosing a particular year or span of years. This can be useful if you are interested in the most recent information about a topic. Other limits include language and you can choose, for example, to include only English articles in the search, or full text so only those available to you as full text are retrieved, and/or patient group which will include child, adult, etc.

Accessing the information

When searching for literature there are a few simple steps that will help you with this process:

- find out what databases are available to you through your education institution or health organization;
- familiarize yourself with these databases and how they work – what subject heading, search filters, truncation and wildcard symbols, etc. are used in each;
- identify your search terms – be exact about what it is you want to find;
- put your search terms into the database you feel is most appropriate, using Boolean terms, truncation, and/or wildcards as appropriate;
- focus, explode, and/or limit your search as appropriate;
- examine the retrieved items for relevant literature – if a particularly relevant article is retrieved, examine its subject headings to identify if you have missed out any relevant areas from your own search.

Once you have practised a few times the process will become easier and you will then find locating relevant literature an easier task.

EBP ACTIVITY

Identify a problem related to your clinical area of practice and using the PICO format generate a question. Using the steps identified above locate three papers relevant to your focus.

SUMMARY

- Four resources are available to make decisions about integrating evidence into practice – systems, synopses, syntheses in the form of systematic reviews and original studies.
- Searching for evidence is a skill that takes time and practice to develop and librarians can be a key resource in finding the information you need.

- It is important to be aware of what resources are available to you when searching for evidence.
- All databases use standard words to describe the content of articles – known as subject headings – and the most well known are the medical subject headings (MeSH terms). Free text and/or MeSH/subject headings can provide the means to locate relevant literature.
- Boolean terms, truncation and wildcards can help you streamline your search and ensure the relevant literature is found.

Further reading

Greenhalgh, T. (2006) *How to Read a Paper: The basics of evidence-based medicine* (3rd edn.) Oxford: Blackwell. Provides an excellent chapter on searching for evidence.

Conclusion to Part 1

The aim of this section was to provide you with an underpinning knowledge of the various aspects of evidence-based practice and the skills associated with the first three aspects of the process as identified in Chapter 1. These are:

- the ability to identify what counts as appropriate evidence;
- forming a question to enable you to find evidence for consideration;
- developing a search strategy;
- finding the evidence.

This section ends with a crossword puzzle, with answers to the clues relevant to Chapters 1, 2, 3 and 4. The answers can be found on page 148.

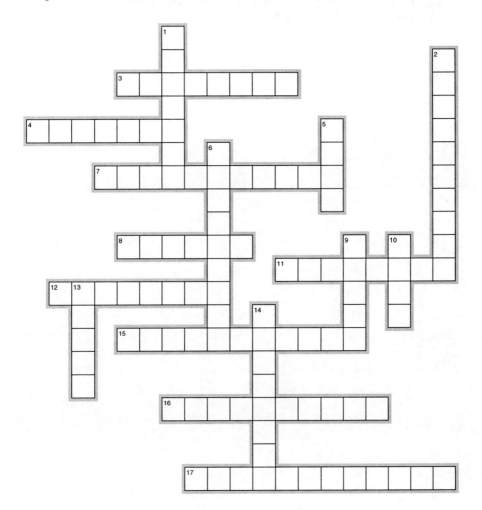

Across

3.   information on which to base best practice
4.   words used to combine search terms
7.   items of evidence grouped together to provide a greater effect
8.   theorist's surname – proposed a framework of nursing knowledge
11. set of logically connected ideas
12. central point for storing information in relation to specific topics
15. considering implications of decisions over time
16. belief that only what can be observed can be called fact
17. belief that humans actively construct their reality

Down

1.   a body of knowledge organized in a systematic way
2.   the belief that reality is ordered and can be studied objectively
5.   terms used to describe medical subject headings
6.   essential aspect of clinical decision-making
9.   knowledge used by practitioners drawn from experience
10. format for creating search questions
13. process for gathering information to promote effective care
14. last name of the 'father' of EBM

Part II

Critiquing the Evidence

What is Critical Appraisal?

Introduction

Critical appraisal is a key component of EBP and as such a core skill for those engaged in EBP. Much of what is written in relation to this area relates to the critical appraisal of published research literature. However, the types of evidence available are increasing, particularly in the form of clinical guidelines. It is essential that you critically appraise all evidence before integrating it into your practice. In this chapter therefore various issues related to critical appraisal and what this means in relation to journal articles and clinical guidelines are considered. Examples of tools that can help you with this process are identified and the skills you need to develop are outlined.

What is critical appraisal?

According to *Collins Dictionary* (1998) the word 'critical' means 'containing careful or analytical evaluation' and appraisal is 'an assessment or estimation of worth, value or quality of a thing'. Therefore critical appraisal can be said to be a careful evaluation of the worth, value or quality of evidence. It is not just about the identifying of weaknesses in a piece of evidence but also about noting the strengths – critical appraisal should be an objective consideration of the merits and limitations of the evidence.

When critically appraising something, Buckingham et al. (2008) suggest there are three central issues to be considered:

1. Validity – do you think the information is trustworthy?
2. Clinical importance – will this information make a difference to the quality/ effectiveness of care?
3. Applicability – is it useable in the practice context?

The end result of critical appraisal should be a balanced consideration of a study's validity and its significance for practice, this will help you make decisions as to how best to incorporate appropriate findings into your practice.

A critical appraisal of the research literature

Parkes et al. (2001: 1) defined critical appraisal as 'the process of assessing and interpreting evidence by systematically considering its validity, results and relevance to an individual's work'. They suggest that a basic understanding of research methods is essential when undertaking critical appraisal. It is therefore important that you develop a basic knowledge of the research process and its various components.

One of the problems with published work is that people assume because something is in print it must be 'good' evidence, but this may not be so. Although most research papers are subject to some sort of peer review process – where other people scrutinize the work and comment on its appropriateness for publication – not all published work is of a good standard. Even when research is of a good quality, most will still have methodological weaknesses, as Nieswiadomy (2008) identified, there is no such thing as a perfect research study as all have flaws or limitations of some sort. If research findings are to be used in practice it is vital you are aware of these limitations and can consider their implications for introducing evidence into your area of practice.

Polit and Beck (2008) have noted that frequently there are 'grey areas' in relation to some aspects of research, with experts having different opinions as to what they believe to be appropriate when conducting a study. As research methodologies develop and studies progress, researchers have to weigh up the differing opinions and issues relating to their area of interest and then make decision about how to proceed with research. This then has an impact on the overall research outcomes. There are often compromises to be made in terms of what is considered ideal and what is practicable in a given situation. These compromises can often relate to issues such as sample sizes, the methods used to collect and analyze data, and/or the interpretation of findings. When critically appraising work you should evaluate these decisions by asking questions such as, 'Would another approach have been better?', 'Does the form of analysis have implications for the findings?' or 'Was the sample size sufficient to justify their conclusions?' and should then decide if these will have implications for the study as a whole and its relevance for your practice.

Issues related to the **validity**, **reliability**, **trustworthiness** and **relevance** of research studies are of prime importance to critical appraisal (D'Auria, 2007) and all of these concepts will be considered in more depth in later chapters. Briefly, however, validity relates to whether or not the claims made in a study are accurate, so for instance if a paper suggests its findings are generalizable, there is a need to consider if the methodology used supports such a claim. Reliability is concerned with identifying if the results are dependable and replicable and involves asking the question 'If the research was repeated would the same results be found?' The concept of trustworthiness relates to whether data can be considered dependable and credible. Finally, relevance is seen as a consideration of whether the findings can be applied to the practice setting. Although these concepts are relevant to all forms of research, different criteria are often needed to make these judgements in relation to different research paradigms.

Quantitative research will tend to be judged in terms of reliability and validity whereas qualitative approaches will generally focus more on **credibility**, **dependability**, **confirmability** and **transferability** (see Chapter 7 for further information). However both sets of criteria are based on the idea of **rigor**, which involves a judgement as to whether the research is of a high quality and whether measures were in place to ensure that the research was conducted in an appropriate way, consistent with the underpinning principles associated with the research paradigm.

Published research papers do tend to have a specific form, being divided in to particular sections. In critical appraisal each of these sections is examined and certain aspects of each section are considered. The format of papers may vary slightly from journal to journal or appear in a different order when certain research approaches are used. However, generally the content remains the same, with all the aspects appearing in some form. This provides a logical approach on which to base your critical appraisal, and Appendix 3 provides a tool containing general criteria to consider when critiquing an article in this way.

ACTIVITY

Identify a topic of interest related to your recent clinical experience. Find two research articles related to this topic – one using a qualitative approach and one using quantitative. Compare the articles' sections, identifying any similarities and differences.

A framework to critique research is offered by Polit and Hungler (1989) which identifies the broad areas that should be considered in critical appraisal which are relevant to all forms of research (see Table 5.1). Parahoo (2006) has argued that the over-arching issues of sources of bias and omissions/exaggeration also need to be considered. Bias is a distortion of the results and/or conclusions and can be

Table 5.1   *Elements for critique*

Dimension	Issues to be considered
Substantive/Theoretical	• Is this an important area to study? • Does it have relevance to practice? • Does it take knowledge in this area forward? • Does the research approach fit with the question to be answered?
Methodological	• Are the research design, sampling method, data collection tool and forms of analysis rigorous and appropriate to the research question/hypothesis?
Practical	• Is the scope of the proposed research too broad? • Have practical issues related to the actually 'doing' of the research been given consideration?
Ethical	• Has the researcher identified the ethical issues associated with the research? • Has ethical approval been sought and given?
Interpretive	• Is the researcher's interpretation of the findings credible in light of the data? • Does the researcher's interpretation appear logical when compared with your own understanding of the area and other research on the topic?
Presentation/style	• Is there enough information? • Is it presented in a clear and concise way? • Are the themes and arguments developed in a logical and reasoned way?

introduced in a number of ways – from the participants, the researcher(s), the methods of data collection, the environment and the phenomena under study. These will be considered in more depth in relation to qualitative and quantitative approaches in the following chapters.

Exaggeration tends to appear in the form of writers overemphasizing the relevance of certain results. For example, if you asked people whether they preferred jam or marmalade on their toast and 46 per cent said jam, you could say almost half of the people questioned preferred jam, or less than half preferred jam, as each statement implies something different in relation to the same result. Omissions will generally fall into two categories – intentional and unintentional. The former will be serious if there is an intention to deceive the reader by deliberately leaving out information that may identify flaws in the work. The latter are the most common and often a result of researchers being so familiar with their work that they forget that others may not have the same level of understanding. This then often results in aspects of a study not being clearly explained or described. Also, in writing for publication researchers will commonly experience problems in terms of article length. Journals allow authors only a fixed number of words which may result in certain aspects being left out or minimal description being included. This is a particular problem in qualitative research where the data collected are generally in the form of words, all of which could not be included in the article.

ACTIVITY

Examine the two papers you chose for the earlier exercise and identify any potential examples of exaggeration and/or omission in these. Consider the implications this might have in relation to the applicability of these studies to practice.

It is important to identify a study's methodology before you begin to critically appraise an article so you can find an appropriate appraisal tool to help with the process. There are a large number of tools available both in books and online. For instance, the NHS Public Health Resource Unit (2007) created a number of tools as part of its Critical Appraisal Skills Programme (CASP) aimed at promoting EBP. CASP tools are currently available to critically appraise:

- systematic reviews;
- RCTs;
- qualitative research;
- economic evaluations;
- cohort studies;
- case control studies;
- diagnostic test studies.

ACTIVITY

Identify the methodological approach used in each of your chosen research studies. Find an appropriate appraisal tool for each of these.

Although qualitative and quantitative approaches are seen as different, they do have some common areas for consideration which are discussed below.

Research design

The research design represents the overall plan for the research and should be coherent and appropriate to the topic under consideration. One particular area for consideration is service user involvement. Just as there is increasing emphasis on the need to ensure service users' voices are heard in the organization and delivery of care, so too is user involvement becoming central to the research process, and this is not simply as participants but rather as part of the whole process. It has been suggested that user involvement can generally occur at three levels (Grant and Ramcharan, 2006):

- consultation – users are consulted in relation to the appropriate issues to be considered and the design of the study;
- collaboration – service users are actively involved in the research process, via recruiting participants, consent issues, collecting data;
- user control – the research is conducted and controlled by service users.

Literature review

A review of the literature relevant to a piece of research will usually be present in some form. It should be up to date, mainly from primary sources, and relevant to the research question/hypothesis and its proposed objective/aims. Parahoo (2006) has suggested four criteria by which to judge a literature review:

1. Does it provide a rationale for the study? The review should identify why it is important the study is undertaken, the benefits and any possible outcomes.
2. Does it put the current study into context? It should consider what is already known about the concepts under consideration and provide a balanced view of the various debates around the chosen focus.
3. Does it provide a review of the research relevant to the topic? Research previously conducted should be considered, any conclusions drawn, and implications for the proposed study identified.
4. Does it provide a conceptual/theoretical framework for the research? As you will see below not all research identifies a theoretical and conceptual framework, however a literature review should provide an overview of the different frameworks available.

Theoretical/conceptual framework

The purpose of research is to generate new knowledge, which involves testing, adjusting and developing theories. Therefore there is a need to identify what theory underpins or how it guides the research being critiqued. The terms 'theoretical framework' and 'conceptual framework' are often used interchangeably, and although there are distinctions between these – the former usually refers to the use of one theory whereas the latter generally entails the combining of concepts from a range of theories – as Parahoo (2006) has pointed out, in practice this distinction is not always recognized by researchers. In fact this aspect is frequently missing from research reports or mentioned only in passing, particularly within quantitative research. It may, however, remain implicit within the literature review, the operational definitions, or the discussion of the finding in relation to other literature.

Ethical issues

The Department of Health (2005: 10) stated that 'the dignity, rights, safety and wellbeing of participants must be the primary consideration in any research study'. All health service research undertaken in UK care organizations has required formal ethical approval since the Research Governance Framework for Health and Social Care (DoH, 2001) became law in 2004. The DoH (2005: 10) requires research involving 'patients, service users, care professionals, volunteers, organs, tissue and data to be reviewed independently to ensure it meets ethical standards'. The regulations governing other countries may vary but the broad principles are generally the same, reflecting the World Medical Association's (2004) Declaration of Helsinki concerning the ethical principles health professionals should consider in undertaking research.

Population

The population is the particular group of people that a researcher is interested in. It could be people with a learning disability who have challenging behaviour or children between the ages of 10 and 16 years who have appendicitis. It refers to the entire group, however data are not usually collected from an entire population.

Sampling

This term describes a segment of the identified population that have been selected to take part in a study. People who form the sample within quantitative research are generally termed **subjects** or **sampling units**. Generally the word **partici- pant** is used in relation to those who take part in qualitative research. This reflects the base philosophy that individuals take an active role in the research process, rather than being passive subjects. Different ways of identifying the sample are used in qualitative and quantitative research and are discussed in more detail in Chapters 6 and 7.

Pilot study

Often before the full research study is carried out, a small 'pilot' study will be con- ducted to test out the design and forms of data collection. This allows for any adjustments to be made to the main study if there are problems with certain aspects. For example, questions in a questionnaire may be changed if they are found to be unclear or ambiguous when tested on a small group first.

Data collection, analysis and results

These areas relate to what type of information is to be collected, and how it will be gathered, processed, analyzed and reported. This will be discussed in more depth in the following chapters.

Discussion

Polit and Beck (2008) have argued that the discussion should address the main findings of the study and what they mean, consider the evidence to support the validity of the findings and examine what limitations may impact on this validity. There is also a need to consider the findings in light of what is already known and to draw conclusions as to the usefulness to practice.

Applicability to practice

Finally, applicability relates to whether research findings can be applied to a setting. To judge applicability sufficient information must be present within the evidence to identify whether the population sampled in the study is comparable with the population identified in a clinical literature review question. Information related to age, cultural beliefs and values, ethnicity and lifestyle is essential if a judgement is to be made. As with any form of research, whilst there may be evidence that a particular treatment is effective there is still a need to consider it in light of specific patient preferences in an area of practice.

Critiquing clinical guidelines

Clinical guidelines are being generated everywhere and now seem readily available on almost any topic. Field and Lohr (1990: 38) have defined guidelines as 'systematically developed statements to assist practitioners and patient decisions about appropriate health care'. Although guidelines have been around for a long time, they have recently become an important aspect of clinical governance and are seen as promoting clinical and cost effectiveness and providing a bridge between research and practice.

Whilst clinical guidelines are a useful aid to increasing the use of research in the delivery and management of care, they do not come problem free. Bugers et al. (2002), for example, reviewed 15 clinical guidelines from 13 countries on Type 2 diabetes. Although there was overall general agreement in terms of management of the disease, some differences in terms of treatment were identified. They found that the guideline recommendations shared little common evidence, with only 1 per cent of the evidence appearing in six or more of the guidelines. This lack of common ground highlights the need to give careful consideration to guidelines before using them in practice. In an effort to remove such differences, processes for guideline development are being generated to ensure that they are produced in a rigorous and appropriate manner (for examples see NICE and National Guideline Clearance).

Sanderlin and AbdulRahhim (2007) have offered guidance for critiquing clinical practice guidelines, suggesting that whilst these are important tools in promoting EBP there are various issues to be considered before implementing them in practice. These relate to:

- the strength of the evidence;
- the objectiveness of approach to the development of guidelines;
- the homogeneous aspect of studies – based on studies that have similar designs and complementary results;
- whether study subjects are significantly similar to the relevant patient group;
- whether the guidelines are based on evidence that has been appropriately appraised.

The Appraisal of Guidelines Research and Evaluation Collaboration (AGREE, 2001) provides a tool for appraising clinical guidelines. This international collaboration's aim is to improve the quality and effectiveness of guidelines by promoting a common approach to the development and assessment of guidelines. The AGREE tool consists of 23 essential items organized into six dimensions for consideration by the appraiser (see Table 5.2 for these criteria). You are asked to score each item using a Likert scoring system, where 4 = strongly agree and 1 = strongly disagree, and to comment on each aspect. The final section asks for a judgement

Table 5.2   *AGREE (2001) Criteria for appraising clinical guidelines*

Scope and purpose

1. The overall objective(s) of the guideline is (are) specifically described.
2. The clinical question(s) covered by the guideline is (are) specifically described.
3. The patients to whom the guideline is meant to apply are specifically described.

Stakeholder involvement

4. The guideline development group includes individuals from all the relevant professional groups.
5. The patients' views and preferences have been sought.
6. The target users of the guideline are clearly defined.
7. The guideline has been piloted among target users.

Rigour of development

8. Systematic methods were used to search for evidence.
9. The criteria for selecting the evidence are clearly described.
10. The methods used for formulating the recommendations are clearly described.
11. The health benefits, side effects and risks have been considered in formulating the recommendations.
12. There is an explicit link between the recommendations and the supporting evidence.
13. The guidance has been externally reviewed by experts prior to publication.
14. A procedure for updating the guideline is provided.

Clarity and presentation

15. The recommendations are clear and unambiguous.
16. The different opinions for management of the condition are clearly presented.
17. Key recommendations are easily identifiable.
18. The guideline is supported with tools for application.

Applicability

19. The potential organizational barriers in applying the recommendation have been discussed.
20. The potential cost implications of applying the recommendations have been considered.
21. The guideline presents key review criteria for monitoring and/or audit processes.

Editorial independence

22. The guideline is editorially independent from the funding body.
23. Conflicts of interest in the guideline in development members have been recorded.

Overall assessment

24. Would you recommend these guidelines for use in practice?

as to the usefulness for practice. The collaboration recommends that a minimum of two people and an optimum of four conduct the appraisals.

The skills of critical appraisal

It is important to remember that the skills of critical appraisal are developed over time, and as with most things the more you practise the easier it will get. Critically appraising something takes time; it shouldn't be a rushed activity as it requires you to read things carefully, checking the information provided, and possibly consulting other people and sources of information.

The first thing to consider is whether the evidence is from a credible source. If it comes from a journal there will generally already be some checks in place – most journals will identify whether or not they subject submissions to peer review. Internet sources do not always have such checks in place – for example, self-publishing sites such as Wikis have little or no control over the information placed on a web page or its trustworthiness. You will need to decide whether you believe a site to be credible, and then check an organization's credentials or ask others what they know about certain sites. This may save you unnecessary work if you later find that a source is not reputable.

Greenhalgh (2006) has suggested beginning the actual appraisal process by 'getting your bearings' and asking three broad questions:

1. What clinical question is being answered?
2. What type of study is it?
3. Is the design appropriate to the area of research?

In asking these questions you can very quickly decide whether or not to continue with your appraisal of a particular piece of evidence. If the evidence doesn't address a question you are interested in, there is no point in continuing. Identifying the type of study will enable you to find an appropriate tool to help you critique the work. The appropriateness of the approach is essential in answering your own clinical question. If you are interested in the effectiveness of an intervention but the approach used is one more suitable to considering the feasibility of using a particular intervention then, once again, there is no point in appraising the study. If the study meets all three of these criteria, then the next step is to undertake a full appraisal.

To critically appraise evidence you initially need to take a step-by-step approach as outlined below, but as your confidence and skills grow you will find you develop your own system.

1. Identify a suitable checklist to use to critically appraise the evidence.
2. Find somewhere quiet where you are unlikely to be interrupted.
3. Read through the paper once, so you have a grasp of the content.
4. Read through it again in more depth, evaluating each part of the paper.
5. Make notes or highlight important bits of the paper as you go along.
6. Have a research book to hand so you can check out information or fill in any gaps in your knowledge as you read.
7. Complete the appraisal and discuss your findings with others.

There are resources available to help develop skills in this area, such as Critical Appraisal Topics (CATs). These are summaries of evidence relating to clinical questions generated in response to specific clinical problems (Foster et al., 2001). Originally a paper-based exercise generated by McMaster University in Canada to encourage medical students to develop critical appraisal skills, CATs created by various individuals are now available online as a possible resource and learning tool for other health professionals. An electronic tool known as a Cat-maker, created by the NHS Research and Development Centre for Evidence-Based Medicine at Oxford, is also freely available to help with the generation of your own CAT. Although this has been developed for the medical profession, the process can also be of use to others in a health-care setting as it can provide a summary of the evidence and ends with a judgement as to its appropriateness to address the question asked.

ACTIVITY

Visit the Centre for Evidence-Based medicine CAT-maker website at http://www.cebm.net/index.aspx?o=1216 and download the tool. Consider whether this would be useful for conducting your own critical appraisals.

CATs are a useful learning tool as they:

- provide an example of critical appraisal in relation to a live issue using accessible evidence sources;
- provide a concise step-by-step method for recording the process of critical appraisal which can then be shared with others;
- help in the development of critical appraisal skills;
- enable a structured and informed approach to clinical decision-making.

However, CATs are not without their disadvantages. They have a limited lifespan unless they are regularly updated and may contain errors due to a lack of individual knowledge or particular forms of interpretation.

In developing the skills associated with critical appraisal it is important to remember that to become proficient takes time and you are not expected to know everything or get it completely right first time. It is important here to know how to find the information you need to conduct the appraisal and to discuss your findings with others and to ask for their opinions.

EBP ACTIVITY

Choose one of the papers you identified earlier. Using the appropriate critical appraisal tool undertake a critical appraisal of this paper, identifying the aspects/ questions you are able to fully critique and those where you need to develop further skills and knowledge. Develop an action plan outlining how you will develop the knowledge and skills you require to complete the task appropriately.

SUMMARY

- Critical appraisal is associated with published research literature, but there is a need to appraise all forms of evidence.
- Critical appraisal should be an objective consideration of the merits and limitations of the evidence.
- Not all published work is of an appropriate standard or applicable to the practice setting, therefore critical appraisal is a key aspect of EBP.
- Critical appraisal skills take time to develop and practice is essential.

Further reading

Crombie, I. K. (1996) *The Pocket Guide to Critical Appraisal*. London: BMJ. Offers a step-by-step approach to critical appraisal and considering appraisals of specific quantitative research approaches.

Parahoo, K. (2006) *Nursing Research: Principles, process and issues* (2nd edn.). Basingstoke: Palgrave MacMillan. Provides an excellent introduction to the research process.

E-resources

Critical Appraisal Skills Programme: provides a range of resources to help with developing the skills associated with EBP. Also provides a range of critical appraisal tools.
www.phru.nhs.uk/Pages/PHD/CASP.htm

National Institute for Clinical Excellence (NICE): provides national guidance on preventing and treating illness and promoting health.
www.nice.org.uk

Netting the evidence: aimed at promoting evidence-based health care, providing resources to support evidence-based activities.
http://www.shef.ac.uk/scharr/ir/netting/

6

Critical Appraisal and Quantitative Research

Learning Outcomes

By the end of the chapter you will be able to:

- provide an overview of quantitative research approaches;
- identify the key areas for consideration when critically appraising quantitative literature;
- debate issues of reliability and validity.

Introduction

Quantitative research is primarily concerned with examining how different things known as variables interact and impact on each other. Florence Nightingale is said to have employed quantitative research methods by collecting statistical data during the Crimean War and saw statistics as a vital tool for ensuring health care was based on sound evidence.

As quantitative research involves 'numbers' and the use of statistics, this often produces a 'panic' response in some people who feel they will not be able to understand the analysis. However, as Greenhalgh (2006) has identified, all you really need to know is what the best test is to apply in given circumstances, what it does and what might affect its validity/appropriateness. It is not necessary to understand the actual calculations involved.

In this chapter I intend to look at the methods used in quantitative research and discuss the issues you should consider when critically appraising. However, it is not my intention to provide a full overview of quantitative research, and for a more in-depth exploration you will need to consider some of the recommended reading at the end of the chapter.

So what is quantitative research?

As identified in Chapter 2, quantitative research has its roots in positivism and in using a deductive approach, starting with a theoretical framework or conceptual

Table 6.1   *Types of variables*

Type	Description
Dependent	• The focus of the research. • The characteristic or behaviour that the researcher is attempting to understand, describe or effect.
Independent	• The factor/characteristic that is considered to have an influence on the dependant variable.
Confounding	• A significant association between two variables occurs because of being associated with a third variable.

model which can predict how things (**variables**) behave in the world. Specific predictions (**hypotheses**) are then deduced from the theory (Polit and Beck, 2008). The aim of quantitative research is therefore to explore the relationships between variables and to test hypotheses. It is seen as using objective, rigorous and systematic approaches. A researcher will identify the variables of interest, clearly define what these are and then usually collect data in a numerical form.

A variable, simply put, is something that varies from one person/situation to another. So weight, temperature, pain, personality traits are all variables. Quantitative research seeks to understand why these variations occur. For example, in mental health depression is a variable as not everyone experiences depression. It is possible to study what factors are linked with the onset of depression. If a variable is extremely varied within a particular group it is said to be heterogeneous and where there is limited variability it is described as being homogeneous. Table 6.1 outlines some different types of variables.

Usually the relationship between *independent variables* and *dependent variables* will be considered. In mental health, for example, you could consider whether age (independent variable) has any implications for the onset of depression (dependent variable). Whether a variable is identified as dependent or independent depends on the focus of the study. In the above example depression is the dependent variable, but you could consider whether depression (independent variable) is associated with suicide (dependent variable).

Polit and Beck (2008) suggest quantitative research generally considers specific questions about relationships, such as:

- the relationship between variables – e.g., is body weight related to the onset of Type 2 diabetes?
- the direction of a relationship between variables – e.g., is someone who is overweight more or less likely to develop Type 2 diabetes?
- the strength of the relationship between variables – e.g., how likely is it that someone who is overweight will develop Type 2 diabetes?
- the cause and effect relationship between the variables – e.g., does being overweight cause the development of Type 2 diabetes?

Usually a hypothesis is generated providing a simple statement of the variables to be considered and the relationship between them. For example I could hypothesize that providing play activities (independent variable) for children prior to surgery will reduce their anxiety (dependent variable).

ACTIVITY

Consider an issue which is causing concern in your area of practice. Identify the variables that might be considered in a study and generate a hypothesis as to the relationship between them.

Usually a large number of people are used in quantitative research, therefore statistical tests are used to help make sense of the data and enable these to be presented in an understandable form. Statistics also help in making judgements regarding the value of research findings for the research population as a whole. Analysis is an attempt to measure the concepts and variables under consideration as accurately and objectively as possible. Objectivity is seen as a central tenet of quantitative research, with the researcher viewed as 'standing outside' of the research process. The intention here is to ensure that neither researcher nor the subjects introduce any form of bias into the research process. Bias is where the results of a study are distorted for some reason (this will be considered in more detail later in the chapter). To reduce bias a process known as *blinding* is often used. Here information relating to the research process is concealed from those on whom the research is conducted and/or those involved in delivering the intervention being studied. For example, if the effectiveness of a particular drug is being tested the experimental group of subjects will receive the drug and the control groups will receive a placebo. The subjects and/or those administering the drug may not be made aware of who is receiving the drug and who is receiving the placebo. If information is withheld from only one of the groups involved – the subjects or those administering the drug – it is called a *single blind study*. If information is withheld from both groups it would be known as a *double-blind study*.

Types of quantitative research

Generally two types of research designs are present within quantitative research:

1. Experimental.
2. Non-experimental.

Experimental approaches, with the most common in a health-care setting being RCTs, actively introduce a treatment or intervention in an attempt to study causal relationships. The aim is to identify whether a particular intervention has an impact on the dependent variable. To be a true experimental design the following three conditions must be met:

- an intervention is controlled by a researcher so some subjects receive the intervention and others don't – this is known as manipulation of the variable;
- at least two groups of subjects are involved – a control group and an experimental group;
- random selection and the allocation of subjects to research groups will occur.

If these three conditions are not all met, the research is described as quasi-experimental, with the most common unmet condition being the random assignment of subjects. Quasi-experimental approaches are used to test the effectiveness of interventions but are seen as less rigorous and often there is less confidence in an ability to generalize the findings.

Concerns have been raised in relation to the quality of the reporting of this type of research. It has been suggested that infrequently the information given is not sufficient to allow for a proper critical appraisal. To address these concerns a number of interested parties (journal editors, researchers, etc.) met together and produced recommendations as to what should be included in reports of RCTs – this is now known as the CONSORT statement (Consolidated Standards of Reporting Trials: see Altman et al., 2001). Most researchers now use this approach in designing and writing up their research studies. This makes critical appraisal much easier as can the use of CONSORT in undertaking this activity. Statements related to other forms of quantitative research are also currently being developed.

ACTIVITY

Visit the CONSORT website at www.consort-statement.org and identify the aspects that are considered to be central to the designing and writing up of RCTs.

Non-experimental qualitative research is used to describe and/or identify associations between variables and would generally be used to address Polit and Beck's first three questions about relationships between variables. However, there is no attempt to manipulate variables or to identify cause and effect relationships. Instead the intention is to observe what is happening without intervening. Often these designs are classified in terms of when the data collection occurs.

Cross-sectional studies will compare different groups within the population of interest, collecting data at a single point in time. For example, if you wanted to measure whether the length of time someone was in residential care impacts on their level of satisfaction, you might collect data at the same point from individuals who had been in residence for three months, six months, nine months and one year and then compare your findings.

Longitudinal studies will collect data at various points over an extended period of time from an identified individual or group of people. For example, if you were interested in the impact of socio-economic factors on the health outcomes of children from birth to age six you would collect data from the same group of children from birth to age six at defined intervals (perhaps every six month for example).

Retrospective studies collect data after an event. For example, patients' notes may be examined for information in relation to a specific treatment and recovery. Alternatively **prospective studies** collect data in relation to a specific independent variable and the dependent variable is measured at a later date. In this approach it

Table 6.2   *Types of quantitative research design*

Experimental	Non-experimental
Pre-test/post-test control group design	Surveys
Post-test-only control group design	Correlation
Solomon four-group design	Comparative
Non-equivalent control group design	Methodological
Times series design	Secondary analysis studies

would be possible, for example, to consider if coping behaviours in relation to stress have an impact on the incidence of myocardial infarctions by measuring stress–coping behaviours in a population and then identifying the number of people who had a myocardial infarction in ten years' time.

The most common types of research design are in the form of **descriptive** and **correlation studies**. Descriptive studies generally observe, describe, and document areas of interest as they occur naturally. Correlation studies are employed to examine the relationships between variables, without any manipulation of the independent variable. Table 6.2 provides a list of the different types of research you are likely to come across.

Critical appraisal

As identified in Chapter 5, there are a number of tools available to help you critically appraise quantitative research. Appendix 4 gives a generic approach to the particular areas to be addressed in this form of critique – those specific to quantitative research are highlighted and an overview is given below. For a discussion of the other general items see Chapter 5. Remember, when critically appraising it is helpful to have good research books to hand so you can check or clarify information as you go along.

ACTIVITY

Find a quantitative research study relevant to your area of practice and an appropriate critical appraisal tool.

Hypothesis/research question and research objectives aims

Not all quantitative research has an hypothesis, particularly descriptive approaches. However, if this is not present there should be a clearly stated research question. If a hypothesis is required this should be a simple statement identifying the relationship between at least two clearly stated variables and should be testable. You will come across different types of hypotheses, including:

- directional – this precisely indicates the nature and direction of the relationship between variables i.e., *positive* (for example, increased physical activity improves mental functioning); or *inverse/negative* (for example, people with learning disabilities display less challenging behaviour when involved in diversional activities); or *difference* (for example, people with depression are more likely to commit suicide than those who are not depressed);
- non-directional – this only identifies that a relationship exists (for example, children differ from adults in the levels of anxiety they experience on admission to hospital);
- null hypothesis – this is where no relationship is identified (for example, there is no relationship between the use of cognitive behavioural therapy and an improvement of mood in people who are depressed).

The aims/objectives of the research should also be clearly identified and reflect the research question and/or hypothesis.

Operational definitions

It is to be expected that concepts used within research will be defined. For example, if a study related to whether wound dressing X is more effective than wound dressing Y in the treatment of leg ulcers, there is a need to define clearly what is meant by wound dressing X and Y, the leg ulcer, the procedures to be used when applying the dressing, and the effects to be measured. Whilst words such as 'leg ulcer' are in common usage, within a research context there is a need to identify precisely what type of leg ulcers is to be considered. Without this information the rigour and the generalizability of the findings can be called into question and the ability to identify if the research is relevant to your own area of practice will be reduced.

ACTIVITY

Read the articles chosen in the above activity. Identify the operational definitions and appraise whether these are sufficiently described to allow you to identify an applicability to your own area of practice.

Data collection methods

The measurement tools selected to collect data should be appropriate to the research question/hypothesis and the operational definitions and should also collect the type and level of data required. Data collection methods in quantitative research can take many forms – questionnaires, observational schedules, self-reporting schedules or bio-physiological measures. All of these approaches involve the measurement of variables through the assignment of numbers to the variables according to the rules specified. For example, there are accepted rules for measuring weight which will allow you to identify clearly what someone weighs and what is the accepted weight range in relation to height and age. However, not all variables will have measures already in place and these then have to be created to allow measurements to be taken.

In considering measurement in quantitative research there is a need to understand:

1. What is being measured.
2. How it is being measured.
3. Why it is being measured in this way.
4. What the rules are in relation to that measurement. (Parahoo, 2006)

Without this information it is not possible to judge whether the data being collected can be trusted and can appropriately represent the focus of the study.

There are two main criteria for assessing research tools – reliability and validity – and both are discussed in more detail below. However, briefly, the reliability of measurement tools relates to the accuracy with which a tool is said to measure the variable, how it is able to reproduce findings consistently and be free from error. Validity relates to whether the tool measures what it is said to measure. Frequently researchers will use tools that have already been tested for reliability and validity. If a new tool is being used then there should be evidence that it has been pre-tested for its reliability/validity.

Data collection protocols are usually produced by quantitative researchers to identify procedures for collecting data. Clear instructions as to what conditions should be met and any specific instruction in relation to the sequencing of collecting and recording information are expected to be present.

Sampling

Studies will almost always involve samples rather than the whole population of interest. If findings are to be generalized to the population of interest, then the sample must be seen as representative of the whole of that population. The sample size required for a particular study is often determined through the use of *power calculations*. Statistical power is the ability of a study to detect statistically significant results. The power of a test is affected by the sample size and power calculations will identify the sample size needed to detect significant differences where they exist. A well-designed study will identify using power calculations for calculating sample sizes.

Quantitative research generally uses what is known as *probability* sampling. In this type of sample every unit within the population of interest has an equal chance of being selected. To ensure representativeness *random selection* procedures are used. Appropriate randomisation is of central importance to a RCT as it is seen as ensuring that neither the researchers nor the subjects will be able to influence the outcomes of a study. Four approaches to probability sampling are available – simple, stratified, systematic and cluster (see Table 6.3).

It is important that clear and precise accounts of the inclusion and exclusion criteria are documented within the study in order that the exact characteristics of the population used for the collection of data are known. Without this information, the generalizability of findings to other client groups will be called into question and therefore this reduces your ability to make decisions as to the applicability of the research to your own area of practice.

Table 6.3   *Types of randomised sampling*

Type	Description
Simple random	• A sampling frame is generated listing all the elements of the population. • A number is allocated to each of the elements. • A table of randomly grouped numbers (computer generated) is used to select sample units for a specified sample size.
Stratified random	• Ensures subgroups (e.g., age, ethnicity, etc.) within a population are present in the sample in the same proportions. • **Proportional stratified sampling** = sample proportions are the same as the population. • **Disproportional sampling** = a large sample of a particular subgroup is needed to consider the relationship between variables in that group. • **Weighting** = adjustments made to statistical analysis to provide the actual population values. • Simple random sampling used to select the subjects from each subgroup.
Cluster random (multi-stage) sampling	• Used in large-scale studies with a widespread geographical population. • Clusters of the target population randomly selected. • Units within each cluster again randomly selected to be part of the sample. • Simple random sampling would be used at each stage.
Systematic random sampling	• Sample units are selected at predetermined intervals e.g., every 5th or 7th or 20th unit on the sampling frame. • Interval used decided by dividing the available target population by the sample size required e.g., 100 units for a sample of 20 = every 5th unit selected (100 ÷ 20 = 5). • Sample frame itself is randomised before using this form of sampling.

Data analysis

Statistical analysis allows quantitative researchers to make sense of the mass of numbers generated in the collection of data. There are four levels of data within quantitative research – nominal, ordinal, interval and ratio (see Box 6.1). The level of data indicates the statistical test to be used. It is beyond the scope of this chapter to give a full account of all forms of data test and analysis and I strongly recommend that you identify a book that you can use to help you understand this aspect of the research process.

Box 6.1   Levels of data

Scale	Description
Nominal	• Simply categorizes groups (e.g., male or female) and assigns a code number to the identifying traits (Male = 1 Female = 2). • Allows the identification of the frequency of a trait within a category – for example, by identifying that 60 per cent of a sample were female.
Ordinal	• Codes information according to an order in relation to specified criteria. • Likert scales produce ordinal data (e.g., strongly agree, agree, disagree, strongly disagree).

(Continued)

(Continued)

Interval   • Rank ordering of characteristics, and the distance between any two
             numbers on the scale is known (e.g., a temperature scale).

Ratio   • Ordering of a trait, the intervals between each rank and the absolute
             magnitude of the trait (e.g., height or weight).

Zellner et al. (2007), having reviewed over 400 research articles in various nursing journals, found that 80 per cent of these used the same ten statistical approaches (see Box 6.2 for a description of these ten approaches). It may be useful to familiarize yourself with these forms of statistical analysis as they are the ones you are most likely to come across.

Box 6.2   Description of 10 statistical tests most commonly used in nursing research

Descriptive statistics

- Mean – *the average sum of a set of values. If the ages of six people were identified as 26, 29 30, 38, 40 and 41, the mean age would be 34 (26+29+30+38+40+41 = 204 ÷ 6 = 34).*
- Frequency distribution – *the arrangement of data in ascending order (lowest to highest value), identifying the number of times a particular value or score occurs. If the stress levels of 50 people prior to surgery were measured and given a numerical score (ranging from 1 to 10) it might result in the following frequency distribution:*

Frequency	2	3	5	8	11	7	6	4	3	1	(n 50)
Score	1	2	3	4	5	6	7	8	9	10	

- Standard deviation – *the average deviation of the values from the mean.*
- Range – *the distance between highest and lowest values which gives a picture of the dispersion of data (a range between 15% and 85% = 70).*
- Percentages, percentiles, and quartiles – *the frequency that something occurs is reported in percentages e.g., 60% of people prefer butter to margarine; a percentile is the point below which a specific percentage of values lies (a score at a 60th percentile means 60% of scores are below that): quartiles divide distribution scores into four equal parts.*

Inferential statistics

- A *t*-test – *examines the difference between the means of two sets of values.*
- Analysis of variant (ANOVA) – *examines the difference between several means.*
- Correlation – *identifies an association between variables where a variation in one is related to a variation in another.*
- Cronbach's alpha – *a reliability index used to measure the internal consistency of a multi-itemed measurement tool, such as an anxiety scale or an assessment tool.*
- A chi square test – *compares data collected in the form of frequencies or percentages.*

Briefly, statistics are identified as being either descriptive or inferential (Box 6.3 identifies the different types of descriptive and inferential statistics). Descriptive statistics, as the term suggests, 'describe' and summarize the data, often in the form of averages and percentages. Within the EBP movement one of the most useful forms of descriptive statistics in decision-making are effect/risk measures. These measures are used to calculate the 'clinical meaningfulness' of findings and are frequently seen in systematic reviews. However, these are also being increasingly included in research reports and it may be useful for you to explore these in more depth (for a brief overview see Chapter 8).

Box 6.3   Types of descriptive and inferential analysis

Descriptive	Inferential	
	Parametric	*Non-parametric*
Frequency	Pearson	chi square
Central tendency (mean, mode, median)	*t*-test	Mann-Whitney
Variability (range and standard deviation)	ANOVA	Spearman rho
Risk (absolute risk, absolute risk reduction, relative risk, relative risk ration, odds ration, numbers needed to treat)		

Inferential statistics allow a researcher to make 'inferences' (draw conclusions) about their findings and are usually divided into two types – parametric and non-parametric. The type of test used usually depends on:

- the sampling method;
- the level of data required (e.g., nominal, etc.);
- the distribution of variables to be measured.

Parametric tests are usually adopted where the sample is randomised, where the level of data is interval or ratio, and where there is a normal distribution of variables. These types of test are generally seen as more powerful than non-parametric tests. Non-parametric tests do not consider a particular form of distribution to be present, and can be used with nominal and ordinal data and also on small samples.

Statistical tests that identify significance – whether an observed result is the product of chance or represents a finding of significance – are based on probability theory. This is commonly referred to as a P value. The smaller the P value the less likely the possibility that the result has occurred by chance. It is usually expressed as $P < 0.05$ (the symbol $<$ identifies it is less than; $>$ would signify more than). Significance levels of 0.05, 0.01 and 0.001 are the most commonly cited P values in relation to the significance of findings. A value of 0.05 identifies that the results are significant at a 5 per cent level, meaning that there is a less than five chances in a hundred (or 1 in 20) likelihood that the result has occurred by chance. A P value of 0.05 is generally accepted as the level at which it is possible to claim a positive result. There are two commonly used tests used to consider significance – *chi-squared* and *t*-tests:

- a *chi-squared* tests the significance between groups;
- a *t*-test identifies the differences between groups.

Where statistical significance is identified confidence intervals are usually calculated to work out how precise the results are. The wider the interval, the less likely the same results would be found if the research was to be repeated a number of times. If you found that wound dressing X improved wound healing in 65 per cent of the sample, there is a need to know how precise that estimate is if it is to be applied to the wider population. The sample result is unlikely to be exactly the same as the population response to treatment. It is possible to calculate an interval (with an upper and lower limit) in relation to the sample result that suggests the range within which the target population response to treatment will fall. If the confidence interval had a lower limit of 25 per cent and a higher limit of 100 per cent, the confidence interval is very wide and therefore the value of 65 per cent is very imprecise. If, however, the confidence interval is between 60 per cent and 70 per cent, the estimate of 65 per cent is more precise and meaningful. Conventionally researchers will usually report confidence intervals of 95 per cent (expressed as 95 per cent CI), which is the range of values (the interval) within which there is 95 per cent confidence that the real value lies for the total population of patients.

Findings

It is usually the norm that descriptive statistics are presented first, to give readers an overview of the variables. Findings are then generally ordered in terms of importance or in relation to the sequencing of the research question/hypotheses. Tables are used where a number of statistical tests are reported. Tables should be presented in a clear and easily understandable manner, with firm links to the written narrative. All data should be accounted for.

Reliability, validity and applicability

Reliability relates to the accuracy of findings and the concern that if the same variables were repeatedly measured in the same way, whether the same results would be reached (Parahoo, 2006). For example, you may be fairly sure that a thermometer will accurately measure your temperature and that it would give the same results if you repeated the measurement at five minute intervals. If two results varied by five degrees, you would question the reliability of the thermometer. In critically appraising research you are considering whether the research design, methodology, and measurement tools have provided accurate findings and if you repeated the research in your own area, whether you could be sure that the same result would be found.

Validity is described by Polit and Beck (2008) as a property of inference. Researchers can only infer that a perceived effect is a result of their hypothesized cause if the research is valid, namely that there is confidence that what was intended to be measured has been measured. Four types of validity are proposed by Polit and Beck:

1. Statistical conclusion validity – where tests are deemed to be appropriate/fair and any identified statistical relationship between the variables is based on sound evidence.
2. Internal validity – where a relationship is proven, that this is the result of the independent variable and not some other circumstances, such as chance, confounding variables, introduction of bias, etc. (see Table 6.4).
3. Construct validity – this relates to the degree a tool measures the thing it is designed to measure. For instance, you may be fairly sure that a thermometer is a valid tool to measure temperature (unless it's broken in some way), but you might be less sure of a tool designed to measure pain.
4. External validity – this concerns the generalizability of findings to other people, and/or settings.

Table 6.5 gives an overview of some of the issues that threaten validity in relation to the above items.

Table 6.4   *Sources of bias*

Type	Description
Selection bias	Inadequate randomization.
Performance bias	Differences in the way an intervention is received/delivered.
Attrition bias	More subjects are lost from one research group than another (control or experimental).
Detection bias	Differences which occur when assessing outcomes or RCTs.
Participant bias	A lack of full disclosure or giving what is considered to be appropriate responses.
Conceptual bias	Faulty conceptualization of a problem, the interpretation of findings or the drawing of conclusions.
Design bias	Faults in any aspect of the research design.
Recall bias	Difficulties relating to the recalling of past events, memory degeneration over time.

Table 6.5   *Factors which may impact on validity*

Type of validity	Threats to validity
Statistical conclusion	• Sample size is small. • Tools lack the precision to measure the variables accurately. • Variations in the implementation of an intervention. • Treatment adherence.
Construct validity	• Hawthorne or placebo effect – people's behaviours as a response to being observed or to the treatment because they believe it will have a positive effect. • Researcher response to subjects encourages certain responses. • Novelty effect – perception of new treatments may result in positive or negative responses from subjects. • Compensation – control group subjects are 'compensated' in some way by health staff or family for not receiving research intervention. • Contamination – control and experimental group receive similar services generally or experimental group member moves to control group by dropping out of the trial.

Validity can also be compromised by confounding variables. As discussed earlier, confounding variables are where a proposed relationship between two variables may actually be due to a third variable. In critically appraising studies you must consider whether a researcher has considered potential confounding variables in the research design and any analysis of the findings.

EBP ACTIVITY

Choose and locate a quantitative article of interest and critically appraise it using the questions in Appendix 4. Identify any aspects where you need to develop further skills and knowledge. Then develop an action plan outlining how you will develop the knowledge and skills you require to complete the task appropriately.

SUMMARY

- The aim of quantitative research is to explore the relationships between variables and test hypotheses. A researcher will identify the variables of interest, clearly define what these are and then collect data, usually in a numerical form.
- The relationship between independent variables and dependent variables is considered. Statistics help in making judgements and generalizations of the value of research findings for a research population as a whole.
- Two types of research designs are present within quantitative research – experimental and non-experimental.
- Quantitative research generally uses what is known as probability sampling.
- There are four levels of data within qualitative research – nominal, ordinal, interval and ratio. The level of data indicates the statistical test to be used.

Further reading

Greenhalgh, T. (2006) *How to Read a Paper: The basics of evidence-based medicine* (3rd edn). Oxford: Blackwell. Provides a number of critical appraisal tools and an easy to read chapter on 'Statistics for the non-statistician'.

Polit, D.F. and Beck, C.T. (2008) *Nursing Research: Generating and assessing evidence for nursing practice* (8th edn). Philadelphia: Lippincott Williams & Wilkins. Gives a good introduction to the various aspects of quantitative research and its approaches.

E-resources

CONSORT website: provides explanations and examples of what is expected to be included in some forms of quantitative research.
www.consort-statement.org

Netting the evidence: aimed at promoting evidence-based health care and providing resources to support evidence-based activities.
http://www.shef.ac.uk/scharr/ir/netting/

Critical Appraisal and Qualitative Research

Introduction

Qualitative research has been used particularly in the social sciences – sociology, psychology, and anthropology – and in many of the health-care professions – nursing, pharmacy and social work. In the past there has been great debate, and at times furious disagreements, about the validity of qualitative approaches which have often been criticized as subjective, biased and lacking in generalizability. In earlier times qualitative and quantitative research approaches have been seen as diametrically opposed. More recently, however, most people would agree that it is important to choose an approach that will provide the most appropriate answer to the question posed. Many research studies now adopt mixed methods, where qualitative and quantitative approaches are used side by side to address the issues under consideration. This chapter considers the methods and approaches used in qualitative research and discusses the issues you should consider when critically appraising literature of this type. However, as with the previous chapter it is not my intention to provide a full overview of the research process, and for a more in-depth explanation you will need to consider some of the recommended reading at the end of the chapter.

So what is qualitative research?

As discussed in Chapter 2, qualitative research represents a different research paradigm to quantitative research. It has different philosophical foundations which give rise to

Table 7.1   *Six basic traits of qualitative research*

Trait	Description
Belief in multiple realities	• There is no one reality/truth. • People actively construct their understanding of the world. • People have different experiences of life. • A number of perspectives are available in relation to any situation/phenomenon.
An understanding of the nature of the phenomena being studied through appropriate methods is provided	• There are multiple ways of understanding various phenomenon. • The most appropriate approach(es) to 'capturing' these understandings must be used. • The phenomenon under consideration dictates the method to be used. • Multiple forms of data collection are often used to ensure a full understanding of the research topic.
Provides an understanding from the subject/participant point of view	• Qualitative research involves developing a theory in relation to a phenomenon – asking questions such as 'what is your experience of caring for someone with a learning disability?'
Research is conducted in the natural environment in which the phenomenon occurs	• No attempt is made to control the environment. • The natural environment provides a way of accessing the participant's perspective whilst in the 'space' that it occurs. • Gives access to any cues or influences on an individual's perspective.
The researcher as part of the process	• Acceptance that all research is conducted in a subjective way. • Researcher is seen as adding to the richness of the data.
Data are said to be 'rich' and 'deep'	• Data are collected in the form of words, describing the perspectives and experiences of the participants.

different ways of thinking about the nature of knowledge and how this can be generated. Qualitative research focuses on words, on how people describe their experiences, perspectives, understandings and beliefs/values. The words collected may be in spoken or written form. Qualitative research is an attempt to provide what is termed as a **thick** or **rich description** of the phenomenon from an **emic** (individual's) perspective rather than an **etic** (outsider's or researcher's) **perspective**. Namely, this is to give a full and thorough account of the research context, the meanings people attach to their experiences, their interpretation of issues and also what motivates them to behave/respond in particular ways. Qualitative research is seen as being holistic, giving a total picture of a phenomenon rather than considering parts in isolation.

It has been suggested that qualitative research has six central traits (Speziale and Carpenter, 2007: see also Table 7.1).

Types of qualitative research

There a number of approaches to qualitative research, each with their own theoretical and philosophical underpinnings. The most common approaches are outlined below and an overview of their various aspects is presented in Table 7.2.

Table 7.2   *Overview of qualitative research approaches*

Approach	Types of research question	Data collection	Example
Phenomenology	Meaning/lived experience	Unstructured interviews	Godfrey, H. (2008) 'Living with a long term urinary catheter: Older people's experiences', *Journal of Advanced Nursing*, 62(2): 180–90.
Grounded theory	Social settings Process questions	Interviews Observation	Coyne, I. & Cowley, S. (2007) 'Challenging the philosophy of partnership with parents: A grounded theory study', *International Journal of Nursing Studies*, 44(6): 893–904.
Ethnography	Culture Beliefs and values	Participant observation Field notes Interviews	Forrester-Jones, R., Barnes, A. (2008) 'On being a girlfriend not a patient: The quest for an acceptable identity among people diagnosed with a severe mental illness', *Journal of Mental Health*, 17(2): 153–72.
Discourse analysis	Verbal interaction What power relationships are present in conversations	Observation Recording of interactions Field notes	Hayter, M. (2007) 'Nurses' discourse in contraception prescribing: An analysis using Foucault's "procedures of exclusion"', *Journal of Advanced Nursing*, 58(4): 358–67.
Action research	Implementing change	Mixed	Vallenga, D. et al. (2008) 'Improving decision-making in caring for people with epilepsy and intellectual disabilities: An action research project', *Journal of Advanced Nursing*, 61(3): 261–72.
Historical	Identifying historical roots and/or practices	Interviews Narratives Documentation	Hallett, C.E. (2007) 'The personal writings of First World War nurses: A study of the interplay of authorial intention and scholarly interpretation', *Nursing Inquiry*, 14(4): 320–9.

Phenomenology

This approach is based in a philosophical tradition developed by Edmund Husserl (1857–1938) and Martin Heidegger (1889–1976), which considers people's everyday experiences. The focus here is on exploring the meaning that people attach to their lived experience and this is closely related to **hermeneutics** which centres on meaning and interpretation – how people interpret their experiences within a specific context. For example, if you wanted to know what it means to someone to be given a cancer diagnosis and how they experience this, you might undertake a phenomenological study.

Grounded theory

Developed by two sociologists, Glaser and Strauss (1967), grounded theory is an approach originally forwarded as a way of developing theories and hypotheses that are 'grounded' in the data collected. Strauss and Corbin (1990) describe a grounded theory as one that 'is discovered, developed, and provisionally verified through systematic data collection and analysis of data pertaining to the phenomenon'. It is based on the idea that human behaviour is developed through people's interactions and their interpretation of these. It is often used to study social processes, considering the changes that occur over time in relation to particular experiences. In nursing it is frequently used to gain an understanding of the process through which people learn to manage and/or adapt to new situations. For example, this approach could be used to consider how children adapt their lives over time following a diagnosis of diabetes.

Ethnography

This research approach has its roots in anthropology, being used to consider the beliefs, values and shared meanings of people in particular cultures. Leininger (1985: 35) defined ethnography as 'the systematic process of observing, detailing, describing, documenting and analysing the lifeways or particular patterns of a culture (or subculture)'. Cultures in this context could relate to an entire social group (such as the culture of people from Romania) or to a small group (such as a particular ward setting). Therefore you could study the beliefs and values of people from Romania in relation to the care of people with learning disabilities. Alternatively you could study how the culture of a particular residential home for people with learning disabilities impacts on the care given.

Action research

Action research can include both qualitative and quantitative approaches and is used to study the effects of actions when these are taken to change or improve something. There are various forms of action research, but the basic tenet is that it is a group activity (Speziale and Carpenter, 2007), usually involving some form of collaboration between the researcher and the participants – practitioners, patients or other stakeholders in the process – with a view to improving/changing practices in a specific area. It is also said to be context bound, in that the research is undertaken because of a defined issue related to a specific area. Its participants are seen as central to decision-making processes and will have the final say as to whether changes are implemented or not. It is often seen as cyclic in nature with problems being identified, changes made, and impacts evaluated.

Discourse analysis

Discourse analysis is relatively new to nursing research and looks at the ways in which people talk about particular issues and the systems people use when communicating with each other. It tries to uncover the rules that govern how people talk about things. Its basic premise is that language is not neutral, and when talking what is said and how it is said will have particular meaning and intentions. Foucault's (1979) work has been particularly influential in this area, focusing on how power is exercised through the use of language. For example, it would be possible to consider what power relations are present when qualified nurses talk to students and what values are present in the language they use.

Historical research

As a research approach, historical methods will collect and interpret historical data in a systematic way. The aim is to provide new insights into a topic area and not to summarize existing knowledge as might be done with a literature review (Speziale and Carpenter, 2007). Generally the form of historical research is underpinned by a particular theoretical framework, such as feminism or postmodernism. Historical research may be in the form of biographical accounts of individuals who can provide oral histories of particular groups. For example, oral histories could be taken from people who have experienced mental health institutions at various points in the twentieth century.

Critical appraisal

As discussed in relation to quantitative research, a number of tools are available to help you critically appraise research and many of these are specifically aimed at qualitative research. (Appendix 5 gives a generic approach to this form of critique, and those areas which are specific to qualitative research are highlighted and discussed below.) The areas that are shared in both qualitative and quantitative research are discussed in Chapter 5. Again, as identified previously having good research books to hand so you can check or clarify information as you go along is crucial to your success.

ACTIVITY

Find a critical appraisal tool for each of the research approaches identified in Table 7.2.

The research question and its aims

Qualitative research will normally have a research question and not an hypothesis, as the intention is to generate understanding in relation to a phenomenon and not to predict a relationship between variables. A research question can take two forms (Cormack, 1996).

1. Interrogative – namely, a statement phrased as a question (e.g., 'What is the lived experience of people admitted to hospital following a suicide attempt?').
2. Declarative – namely, a statement which 'declares' the purpose of the study (e.g., 'It is intended to study the experience of people admitted to hospital following a suicide attempt').

The best research questions are short and clearly identify a specific area of study. A question should set the scene for the research design that will allow that question to be answered. Some researchers will pose a series of questions, others will identify a series of aims in relation to the question asked. The research question and aims should have the same intentions.

Literature review

An extensive literature review is not always the starting point for qualitative research. Often only sufficient literature to provide a focus for the study will be considered. In phenomenological research the literature may not be reviewed until after the data have been collected and analyzed. In grounded theory the literature is reviewed at various points throughout the data collection process and is used as a comparison for the interim research finding. This lack of initial literature review is to ensure that the analysis of the data is not influenced by what is already known about a topic. However, there is an expectation that the findings will be considered in light of the available literature, so that the study can be compared with other work and any issues regarding the transferability of findings to other settings can be identified.

Where a literature review is provided, the criteria identified by Parahoo (2006) as described in Chapter 5 (see p. 58) can be applied.

Methodology

The chosen methodology should enable the research question to be answered. If the question asks about the meaning of something or an individual's experience, then you would expect to see a phenomenological design. If the stated aim is to investigate issues related to culture – beliefs, values, social norms – then an ethnographic approach would be more appropriate. There should be a match between what the researcher wants to know and the methodology used to answer the question. Table 7.2 will give you an idea of the methodologies expected to be seen in relation to particular areas of study.

Reflexivity

Whilst researcher involvement in the research process is a central tenet of qualitative research, there is an expectation that a researcher will discuss their beliefs, values, ideas and personal biases relating to the topic they are exploring and this is usually done in the form of a reflective account. This reflexivity is seen as having two purposes. Firstly, it makes the investigator aware of how their own beliefs may influence the data collection and interpretation. Having explored their own perspectives it is normally expected that the researcher will put aside their beliefs in what is termed as **bracketing**. Here the researcher is expected not to make judgements about the appropriateness of what they see or hear, instead being open to what the data reveal rather than imposing their own beliefs on what is collected. The second aspect relates to acknowledging that the researcher is part of the research process and ensures that readers are aware of this.

ACTIVITY

Identify an area you would be interested in researching. Write a short reflective piece identifying what beliefs and values you have in relation to the area and how these might impact on any research you chose to undertake.

However, whilst this process is an integral part of qualitative research the reflective account will often be missing from published work. The word limits imposed by journal publishers on authors of papers frequently result in this aspect being left out. When this is the case, the only insight given into researchers' perspectives and backgrounds in terms of the research phenomenon will be gained through examining their qualifications and job titles as given at the beginning of the article.

Ethical issues

As identified in Chapter 5, all health service research requires ethical approval, however the nature of qualitative research will bring a distinct set of ethical issues into sharp relief. The interpersonal nature of most qualitative research (i.e., that the research and the participants are in direct contact and form a close, albeit brief, trusting relationship) requires researchers to be aware of any possible emotional impact that research may have on participants. Speziale and Carpenter (2007) highlighted that various aspects are important in qualitative research and are as such areas you should consider when critically appraising.

1. *Informed consent* – within qualitative research participants must be allowed to withdraw this consent at any point. 'Process informed' consent is often adopted: here a participant's consent will be re-evaluated at various points within the study and their involvement stopped if necessary.
2. *Confidentiality and anonymity* – the one-to-one interaction between participant and researcher means that anonymity is not possible in the same way as in quantitative research: the researcher will obviously know where the data came from. However, confidentiality can and must be maintained with every effort made to ensure that any participants are not recognizable in the data used to support the descriptions of results.

3. *The researcher–participant relationship* – the researcher must be clear about the boundaries of this relationship. This is a particular issue for a health-care professional, who may find their role as care provider conflicting with their role of researcher.
4. *Sensitive issues* – some of the issues discussed during data collection can be distressing for participants and/or researchers. It is important that a researcher identifies mechanisms for dealing with such issues and how participants will be supported following data collection.

ACTIVITY

Imagine you are conducting a research study discussing a topic which may cause the participants to become distressed. What support do you think it would be important to offer to them.

Sampling/participant selection

Individuals will usually be selected to participate in particular research because they will have had experience or are involved in the phenomenon being studied. For instance, if the research question is 'What is the lived experience of people with schizophrenia?' people selected to participate in a study would be those with schizophrenia, as only they would be able to describe their experiences.

As the intention with qualitative research is to gain a greater understanding of an area of interest, not to generalize findings, randomised sampling is not an issue here. There are various approaches to sampling a population of interest:

- convenience – the most conveniently available people are selected, those who are closest to hand and relevant to the phenomenon of interest;
- snowballing – a form of convenience sampling where having identified an informant to tell you about a phenomenon, they then identify someone else;
- purposive or purposeful – selecting people who can tell you about the research phenomenon: this approach tends to be used in phenomenological studies;
- theoretical – a framework is created in which the principal concepts related to the study are identified and individuals are selected to participate who are judged to have theoretical purpose/relevance. The researcher clearly states the basic types of participants to be included and how these individuals will facilitate the collecting of appropriate data to describe the phenomenon. This approach is most often seen in grounded theory.

Sample sizes in qualitative research are normally small in comparison to quantitative research. It is not unusual to see research conducted on ten people only. The nature of the data collected and subsequent analysis makes large samples almost impossible to handle. For example, one 45-minute interview can produce 30 pages of transcribed information. If you have just ten participants this would result in 300 pages requiring analysis. The aim of qualitative research is to reduce this huge amount of information to a manageable size without losing the intended meaning of the participants.

Table 7.3   *Types of data collection*

Type	Description
Interviews	• Unstructured – no pre-prepared questions apart from asking participants to talk about the phenomenon of interest. • Semi-structured – a guide to asking open questions related to the areas of interest prepared in advance. • (Structure – not used in qualitative research.)
Focus groups	• Group interviews – 6 to 12 people discussing a topic.
Observation	• Participant observation – the research is part of the group and is involved in its activities. • Observer-participant – the researcher generally observes and may interview members of the group and also may participate in some activities. • Complete observer – no interaction between observer and participant.
Field notes	• In ethnography these involve the documenting of observations and narratives. • In phenomenology these may involve the recording of individual expressions and other aspects not captured with the audio recording of interviews.
Diaries	• Unstructured – where people are asked simply to record their thoughts and feelings. • Structured – where people are asked to write about specific aspects.
Documentation	• Patient notes, historical records, health service documentation and records, published and unpublished works.

The sample size is largely decided by the type of research, the quality of the information provided by the participants and the sampling approach used. Often qualitative researchers will talk about reaching **data saturation**, particularly in grounded theory. This is the point where no new information is being collected from participants and is also usually the point where the data collection will stop. So for example, if data saturation is reached after interviewing 12 people then no further interviews will be conducted.

Data collection

There are various forms of data collection available to the qualitative researcher, but all of them involve the collection of 'words' in some shape or form. Table 7.3 provides an overview of the main types of activity. In appraising a study it is important to consider whether the form of data collection used will provide the researcher with the most appropriate data.

It is essential that a study identifies how the information from participants was recorded. Many researchers will use audio recording devices and some may incorporate video recording to ensure that actual responses are captured. Whilst field notes are useful and can add to the picture they do tend to be incomplete and therefore will not enable researchers to revisit the interaction in its original form.

Data analysis

Polit and Beck (2008) proposed that qualitative data analysis is more difficult than quantitative analysis to do but easier to understand, which is a bonus for those who are critiquing rather than doing the research. However, it is not always easy to fully appraise the findings as you cannot know if the authors have given an appropriate representation of their participants' stories.

All qualitative analysis involves some sort of content analysis where researchers will create categories and themes from the data. As these categories are created, a coding system is then developed which allows statements made by participants to be grouped together in particular categories. Once such categories have been identified these may then be grouped further into themes. Data can be handled manually or analyzed using computer assisted qualitative data analysis systems (CAQDAS), such as ATLAS/TI and Nvivo. However, as there are a number of approaches to qualitative research the content analysis can take various forms. Note this lack of a universal approach can make it difficult for you to critically appraise the work.

When critically appraising a qualitative analysis you must look to see whether the author has given you enough information to make a judgement as to whether the analysis has been conducted in an appropriate way. There are a number of basic tenets you would expect to see described.

1. Data transcription – how the data are translated from audio to a written form; what steps were taken to ensure the data were best quality, including an identification of any problems related to transcription (e.g., background noise, poor tape quality, participant's voice inaudible).
2. Identification of the tool used for analysis – a number of tools would be available and the one chosen should be appropriate to the research methodology. For example, you would not expect a grounded theory methodology to include Colaizzi's (1978) approach which is specific to phenomenology. The researcher involved should clearly identify the approach taken and you should be able to follow this step by step through the paper.
3. Interpretation – this occurs at the same time as the analysis, as the researcher reads and re-reads the data and then codes, categorises/themes and tries to make sense of that data. The author should give details of how the interpretation was arrived at.

ACTIVITY

Find three different examples of tools that can be used in the analysis of qualitative data.

Issues of rigour

As Speziale and Carpenter (2007: 48) have pointed out, decisions as to the rigour of a particular research study are often a 'judgement call'. They go on to suggest that two fundamental characteristics of qualitative research should be present when making this judgement as to whether it meets the implicit goal of providing an accurate account of the participants' perspective.

1. Is there adequate attention paid to the collection of information?
2. Is there confirmation of the accuracy of the information?

Table 7.4   *Criteria for assessing the rigor of qualitative research*

Criteria	Ways of identifying if criteria are met
Credibility	• Findings returned to participants for confirmation that they are a true representation of their experiences. • All data are accounted for, including instances where the data are inconsistent with other findings. • Triangulation.
Dependability	• Reporting of unexpected events and how these were dealt with. • Recording methods ensured quality of data. • Triangulation.
Confirmability	• Evidence of reflexivity. • Provision of an 'audit trail' to enable the thought and decision-making processes to be identified (a research diary or recording mechanisms within CAQDAS).
Transferability	• Providing a full description of the research setting and participants. • Identifying that the findings have relevance to similar situations. • Theoretical triangulation.
Authenticity	• The reality of the participants' lives is conveyed, enabling you to understand the range of feelings experienced by those involved.

An alternative way for considering the rigor of qualitative research is provided by Lincoln and Guba (1985) and Guba and Lincoln (1994). Table 7.4 provides an overview of the proposed criteria.

Triangulation is a strategy used in qualitative research to ensure that the approach has rigor and increases the credibility of results. The idea comes from a navigation term used to describe how sailors or pilots plot the location of their ship/plane. Imagine you are on a boat in the middle of the ocean and you know the location of the lighthouse in the distance and an island to the west. Using a compass you take bearing readings (the angle between the lighthouse and North on the compass, and the island and the North point) and find this to be 20 degrees and 360 degrees respectively. You then plot each line on a map and if the readings are correct the lines should intersect at a certain point identifying your position (see Figure 7.1).

Triangulation in qualitative research is based on the idea that the phenomenon of interest can be 'plotted' from different angles so a clearer description of it is given. Four types of triangulation are possible (Denzin, 1989):

1. Data triangulation – where more than one source of data is collected. This can be done in three ways:

    i.   Time – collecting data at different points in time: for instance, you might interview people at intervals of three, six and 12 months in relation to a particular phenomenon.
    ii. Space – collecting data from different sites: perhaps including different in-patient units in a study.
    iii. Person – collecting information from different groups of people: for example, interviewing nurses on Bands 5, 6 and 7, or service users and their carers.

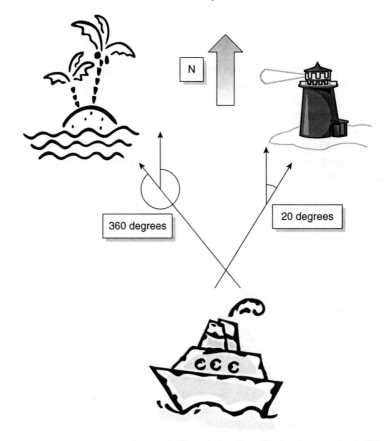

Figure 7.1   *Triangulation – where the lines cross marks the location of the boat*

2. Methodological triangulation – here two or more research methods are used in:
   i.   The research design – for example, combining qualitative and quantitative approaches.
   ii. The data collection techniques – for example, using diaries and interviews.
3. Investigator triangulation – here two or more investigators, each having their own specific area of expertise, will collect, analyze and interpret the data.
4. Theoretical triangulation – having more than one theory underpinning the analysis of the data. As the data are analyzed they are viewed through the 'lens' of different theories to see if alternative interpretations will arise from examining these in multiple ways.

EBP ACTIVITY

Choose one of the research articles identified in Table 7.2 and critically appraise it using the questions in Appendix 4. Identify the aspects/questions where you need to develop further skills and knowledge. Then develop an action plan outlining how you will develop the knowledge and skills you require to complete the task appropriately.

SUMMARY

- There are a number of approaches to qualitative research, each with their own underpinning theoretical and philosophical aspects, generally focusing on how people describe their experiences, perspectives, understandings and beliefs/values.
- Ethical issues take a particular form in qualitative research.
- Sample sizes in qualitative research are normally small in comparison to quantitative research. Individuals are usually selected to participate in particular research because they have experience or are involved in the phenomenon being studied.
- There are various forms of data collection available to qualitative research, but most of these involve the collecting of 'words' in some shape or form and analysis includes some sort of content analysis where researchers will create categories and themes from the data.

Further reading

Spezial, H.J.S. and Carpenter, D.R. (2007) *Qualitative Research in Nursing* (4th edn). Philadelphia: Lippincott Williams & Wilkins. Provides an overview of various aspects of qualitative research, with different approaches and guidelines to help in the critical appraisal of different methods.

Polit, D.F. and Beck, C.T. (2008) *Nursing research: Generating and assessing evidence for nursing practice* (8th edn). Philadelphia: Lippincott Williams & Wilkins. Gives a good introduction to the various aspects of qualitative research and its approaches.

E-resources

Critical Appraisal Skills Programme: provides a range of resources to help with developing the skills associated with EBP. Also provides a range of critical appraisal tools.
www.phru.nhs.uk/Pages/PHD/CASP.htm

Netting the evidence: aimed at promoting evidence-based health care and providing resources to support evidence-based activities.
http://www.shef.ac.uk/scharr/ir/netting/

Systematic Reviews and Evidence-Based Practice

Introduction

The explosion of literature related to health care has made it almost impossible for any practitioner to keep abreast with all current research findings. David Sackett (2008) stated that to keep up to date in his speciality he would need to read at least 17 papers a day, every day of the year. **Systematic reviews** (SRs) provide a rigorous review of research findings in relation to specific questions, saving practitioners the time and effort it would take to search and appraise a large body of evidence. Whilst it is not expected of health professionals in general that they undertake SRs (these can be both complex and time-consuming to complete), there is a need to be able to appraise them and to evaluate the usefulness of their findings for practice.

Pearson et al. (2007) see systematic reviews as fundamental to EBP, providing practitioners with sound evidence on which to base their practice. SR is often a term that is used interchangeably with **meta-analysis**, but as you will see from the discussion below the two are not the same – the latter can be part of the former but is not always present. SRs have been primarily associated with quantitative research, but increasingly systematic reviews of qualitative research are being undertaken with an accompanying **meta-synthesis** of the qualitative findings. There are some SRs which consider both qualitative and quantitative studies and provide both a meta-analysis and a meta-synthesis of relevant studies. As SRs can give an overview of primary research they can be of immense use in clinical practice.

The processes involved in systematic review can seem a little overwhelming to the novice appraiser, however if these are considered in a step-by-step way it is possible to gain a picture of whether a review will be applicable to your own area of practice. This chapter will consider the methods and approaches used in SRs and the areas to be considered when critically appraising this form of evidence.

What is a systematic review?

As identified in Chapter 1, in many ways EBP can be seen as having its origins in Professor Archie Cochrane's criticisms of the medical profession for its failure to use the body of evidence available to it in an appropriate way. Prior to the emergence of EBP summaries of studies more frequently appeared in a form which Greenhalgh (2006) terms 'journalistic reviews'. Here papers were reviewed, selected and analyzed in an ad hoc manner, subject to the vagaries of the person conducting the literature review. In many ways this left any interpretation provided open to accusations of bias and the lack of a systematic approach gave readers little evidence on which to consider the credibility of the findings. However, since the advent of EBP, SRs have become more prevalent and are generally conducted using rigorous designs, often adhering to a standard format or at the very least one that is made explicit and is reproducible. For example, to improve the reporting of meta-analyses a statement has been designed similar to the CONSORT framework for RCTs discussed in Chapter 6. Known as QUOROM (Quality of Reporting of Meta-analyses), this identifies what should be included and considered when designing and writing up meta-analyses. Many meta-analyses now follow the structure provided by this QUOROM statement.

ACTIVITY

Locate and read the following article by D. Moher et al. (1999): 'Improving the quality of reports of meta-analyses of randomised control trials: The QUOROM statement', *The Lancet*, 254: 1896–1900. Identify two of the aspects discussed in relation to meta-analysis that you feel you know least about. Then draw up and implement an action plan to develop your learning in relation to these two aspects.

Systematic reviews are a form of research, often termed as **secondary research** as secondary sources of data are used – usually coming from primary research that has collected data from an original source (participants, subjects, etc). As the Cochrane Collaboration identifies, SRs 'seek to collate all evidence that fits pre-specified eligibility criteria in order to address a specific research question'. The process of 'collating' this evidence is a systematic process (Box 8.1 identifies the steps associated with SRs). Pearson et al. (2007) have added a further step which involves the creation of a best practice guide based on the evidence identified in the systematic review. As you can see these are very similar to the steps identified in relation to EBP.

Box 8.1   Systematic review process

Formulate question, aim, and outcomes
Define the terms
Identify the inclusion/exclusion criteria
Identify the search strategy
Search the literature
Appraise the evidence
Synthesize the data where appropriate or provide a narrative account of findings
Conclude and make recommendations

Types of systematic review

There are two main types of systematic review – qualitative and quantitative. The basic steps for each are the same, however differences occur in the data extraction and summarizing. Whilst in both types of SR the reviewer is 'pooling' the results from 'like' studies and creating a larger data set for analysis (Pearson et al., 2007), the underpinning philosophies and methods used are different. The pooling of quantitative data is seen as aggregating the findings, while the pooling of qualitative findings can be an aggregation or interpretation of the findings depending on the approach used. A meta-analysis can also be seen as giving a picture of the effectiveness of an intervention, while meta-synthesis increases the understanding of a phenomenon of interest. Where statistical data are the focus a meta-analysis may be conducted. If the data are qualitative in nature then a meta-synthesis will be undertaken. A number of tools are readily available (see Box 8.2).

Box 8.2   Electronic tools for data extraction and synthesis

Review Manager	Commonly know as 'rev-man', created by the Cochrane Collaboration for systematic reviews of effectiveness studies.
Systems for the Unified Management of the Assessment & Review of Information (SUMARI)	Created by JBI, this is a collection of tools to enable the systematic review of various types of evidence: • MAStAri – effectiveness studies. • ACTURI – economic studies. • QARI – qualitative studies. • NOTARI – text, expert opinion and discourses.

Meta-analysis is defined by Greenhalgh (2006: 122) as 'a statistical synthesis of the numerical results of several trails which all address the same question'. It enables the bringing together of results for studies that are said to be homogeneous in nature – considering the same outcome of the same intervention on the same population – in an objective way. The power to detect relationships between

Table 8.1   *Meta-synthesis approaches*

Approach	Description	Example
Nolbit & Hare (Meta-ethnography)	• Considers how studies relate to each other (either seen as being reciprocal – comparable – or refutational – in opposition). • Translates studies, ensuring the main concepts are reflected. • Synthesizes the various translations into a comprehensible whole. • Provides a narrative account of the synthesis.	Hildingh, C. Frindlund, B. & Lidell, E. (2007) 'Women's experiences of recovery after myocardial infarction: A meta-synthesis', *Heart and Lung*, 36 (6): 410–17.
Paterson et al.	Three components: • Meta-data analysis – analysis of the findings. • Meta-method – the rigour with which each study is conducted is incorporated into the meta-synthesis. • Meta-theory – the studies' theoretical underpinnings are analyzed. • These three components are brought together to produce a meta-synthesis of findings.	Lloyd Jones, M. (2005) 'Role development and effective practice in specialist and advanced practice in acute hospital settings: Systematic review and meta synthesis', *Journal of Advanced Nursing*, 49 (2): 191–209.
Sandelowski & Barroso	• An integration of the findings. • Integrates interpretation into a new description of the phenomenon of interest.	Sandelowski, M., Lambe, C. & Barroso, J. (2004) 'Stigma in HIV-positive women', *Journal of Nursing Scholarship*, 36 (2): 122–8.

variables is increased due to the increased sample size created through combining studies. This in turn allows conclusions to be drawn about the size of the effect of an intervention.

Meta-synthesis is a growing area of interest, but it is not without its dissenters. Heated debate exists around whether the meta-synthesis of qualitative findings is appropriate or indeed possible. For those who advocate meta-synthesis, some would propose that only findings from studies using the same methodology (phenomenology, ethnography, etc) are possible, whilst others would argue that it is possible and appropriate to combine the findings from various methodologies. Polit and Beck (2008) have highlighted three approaches to meta-synthesis – Noblit and Hare's; Paterson, Thorne, Can and Joilling's; and Sandelowski and Barroso's. The main aspects of these are identified in Table 8.1.

The generalizability of qualitative meta-syntheses is also hotly debated. As qualitative research itself makes no claims to generalizability, with the emphasis being seen as providing thick description and insight into a phenomenon, there are concerns about making such claims in relation to the meta-synthesis of results. Nevertheless, the pulling together of 'like' studies and providing a wider consideration of a particular phenomenon in relation to a particular group can have its practical uses.

Critiquing a systematic review

As identified in Chapter 5, there are a number of tools available to help you critically appraise. (Appendix 6 gives a generic approach to particular areas to be addressed in critically appraising systematic reviews.) As always, when critically appraising it is helpful to have good research books to hand so you can check or clarify information as you go along.

> ## ACTIVITY
>
> Find one tool suitable for critically appraising a meta-analysis and another for a meta-synthesis.

Question, objectives and inclusion criteria

All systematic reviews should have a clearly identifiable question generally present in the PICO format or a variation of this. Without this the reviewer and the reader will not be able to decide which are the relevant papers to be included and which should be rejected. While a particular question, such as 'Does eating breakfast improve cognitive functioning in children?', may initially sound appropriate, when you start to pull it apart and consider each aspect – such as what is meant by children (all under-18s or a specific group?), breakfast (a slice of toast or a 'full English'?) and cognitive functioning (alertness, memory, understanding, completion of tests?). Then it becomes apparent that the need for a clear identification of the various facets is central to the whole process.

As with any research, objectives should be clearly stated and should flow from the question. The inclusion criteria will identify the limits of the review and give a clear indication of what is to be included in the review and what is not. Sound justifications are expected to be present for the setting of such limits as well as a clear exploration of the implications of these for the review.

Searching for the literature

The methodology used to identify the literature relevant to a particular SR is a central issue when judging the rigour of a SR. As Pearson et al. (2007) have pointed out, the quality of the SR is reduced if the search strategy is poorly designed and implemented. In undertaking a review, a reviewer must be sure that all studies relevant to a topic are identified. This often requires a complex search strategy in which the search terms are clearly identified, thus ensuring that any literature relevant to the review is located. The same principles discussed in Chapter 4 will apply in identifying what terms are appropriate.

In searching the literature it is expected that:

- all relevant electronic databases are included;
- the hand searching of printed journals is undertaken;
- reference lists are checked for potential sources;
- grey literature is considered;
- raw data and other unpublished sources generated through personal communications are included where appropriate.

In critically appraising a SR it is important to consider if all relevant sources of literature have been included as this may have an impact on the rigour of the review.

ACTIVITY

List any databases and other sources of information which you would consider key to finding literature related to your own central area of practice.

Quality assessment

The quality of the evidence to be included in the review will generally be assessed and some form of critical appraisal of each study will be undertaken. Therefore the tool used for this appraisal should be identified and appropriate to the type of research under consideration. In undertaking this appraisal, the Cochrane Collaboration advocate the weighting of those studies included in terms of strength – the stronger the study, the greater the weight it is given in the meta-analysis. The Joanna Briggs Institute advocates rejecting those studies identified as not being of an appropriate standard.

The use of two critical appraisers is the norm in SRs. These appraisers act independently, subjecting each piece of evidence for inclusion in the SR to a robust appraisal process. The two will then confer and reach an agreement as to the quality of each individual study for inclusion in the review.

Data extraction

The form of data extraction should be clearly identified. Various tools are available to assist with the extraction data (see Box 8.2). For quantitative reviews, the initial information should be apparent in relation to the studies and is usually presented in the form of tables identifying:

- each study's inclusion criteria;
- the sample base and drop-out rates;
- patients' characteristics – e.g., age, gender, ethnicity;
- the intervention – details of the exact form of intervention and how it was delivered (e.g., routes, dosages, timing, instructions for delivery);
- the outcome measures – the reviewer should clearly identify what outcome measures are under consideration;
- the results.

In relation to qualitative reviews, it is expected that a study's methodology (phenomenology, ethnography, etc), cultural features (age, socio-economic group, and ethnicity) and form of data collection (interview, focus group, etc) will be clearly highlighted.

These tables will allow you to compare various studies and help you to make a judgement as to the rigour of the SR. If this table indicates there is significant heterogeneity within the studies then it is unlikely that the results of the study will be subjected to meta-analysis. It is possible to conduct a meta-synthesis of heterogeneous qualitative studies and this is discussed later in the chapter.

Summarizing the evidence

It is not always possible or appropriate to pool data in the form of meta-analysis and in such cases a narrative integration, a written summarizing of the findings, will be provided. The narrative should be clear, concise and give a coherent description of the data.

ACTIVITY

Locate the following article which provides a narrative summary of the findings. If there are aspects of the information which you do not have sufficient knowledge to appraise, create an action plan identifying how you will develop this knowledge.

Bee, P., Playle, J., Lovell, K., Barnes, P., Gray, R. and Keeley, P. et al. (2007) 'Service users' views and expectations of UK registered mental health nurses: A systematic review of empirical research', *International Journal of Nursing Studies*, 45: 442–57.

Meta-analysis

Greenhalgh (2006) has suggested that the mere term 'meta-analysis' strikes fear into the hearts of many students and practitioners, being seen as a statistical analysis of statistical analyses. However, as Greenhalgh advocates, often the meta-analysis is easier to understand than the original statistics. Akobeng (2005) proposed meta-analysis should have two parts:

1. Calculating a measure of treatment effect (common measures are odds ratios, relative risk and risk differences – see Table 8.2) and the confidence interval for each study.
2. Calculating the overall treatment effect.

The reviewer begins by deciding which of the outcome measures of the studies reviewed are to be used for the meta-analysis – in most studies a number of outcomes will be measured, although only some of these may be of interest to the reviewer. The findings in relation to these outcomes are then presented as treatment effect measures which can identify the strength and direction of the relationship between the independent and dependent variables.

Table 8.2   *Treatment effect measures*

Measure	Description
Odds ration	Measures ratio of the odds of an outcome in the intervention group to the odds of the outcome in the control group. One = no difference between groups. Undesirable outcomes; less than one = intervention effective in reducing risk.
Relative Risk (RR)	Measures the ratio of risk in the intervention group to that in the control group. RR of 1.0 = no difference between the groups.
Risk Difference (RD)	The absolute difference in the outcome rate in the groups. RD 0 = no difference between groups.
Absolute Risk Reduction (ARR)	The difference in event rates between the control group and the treatment group.
Numbers Needed to Treat (NNT)	The number of people who need to be treated to prevent one undesirable outcome.

The reviewer will also identify what is known as statistical heterogeneity –
that is, how diverse the effects are across the various studies. This is usually
demonstrated through the use of forest plot graphs, sometimes referred to as
'blobbograms' (see Figure 8.1 for an example). Each horizontal line is the
confidence interval for an individual study. The symbol or 'blob' in the
middle of each line is the estimated treatment effect of the study (odds
ratio, relative risk, etc): the size of the blob represents the size of the effect.
The width of the line represents the 95 per cent confidence interval of this
treatment effect – as identified in Chapter 6, the wider the interval the less
precise the estimate. The black line down the middle is the 'line of no effect'.
In this example if the confidence interval of a particular study crosses the 'line
of effect' it means either there is no significant difference between treatment
groups and/or the sample is too small to be confident that that there is an
effect. The heterogeneity of studies can be instantly assessed in forest plot
graphs as the more scattered the lines the more heterogeneous the results. The

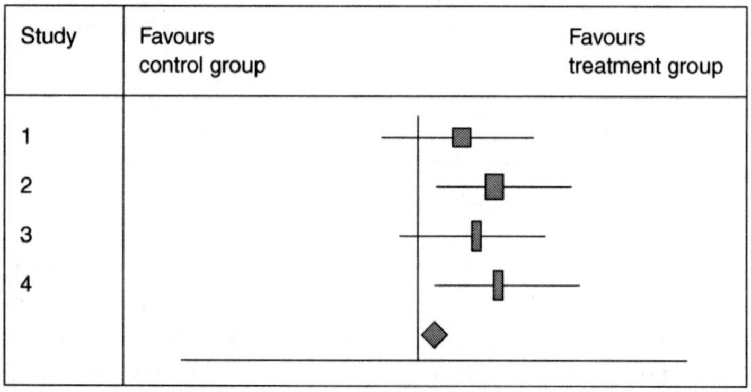

Figure 8.1   *Forest plot graphs*

more heterogeneous the results the less confidence there will be in the ability to use these results in practice.

The diamond below all the horizontal lines represents the pooled effect of the data. Where this is placed reflects whether overall there is confidence that one treatment is better than the other. On the line means that for the average person there is little choice between the two, while to the left of the line identifies that one is indeed better than the other.

If studies are seen as homogeneous and a heterogeneity of treatment effects is identified between studies, Khan et al. (2003) suggest that this may due to differences in the characteristics of:

- the population;
- interventions;
- outcomes;
- the study design.

For example, if in one study the sample of older people included the 'young old' (between the ages of 65 and 80 years of age) and in another the sample was made up of 'old older' people (80 years old+) that would represent a heterogeneous population and would explain why differences in the effect of an intervention were seen. Where none of the above is apparent, Khan et al. suggest that heterogeneity may be a result of **publication bias**. This type of bias occurs due to a tendency in some areas for only positive results to be published, and in using such findings for SRs a bias towards effectiveness is likely. It is expected that reviewers will explore this possibility.

Frequently in meta-analysis it can be seen that where a number of trails have reported no significance, the pooled data will result in a statistical significance. The Cochrane symbol is a representation of the most famous incidence of this pooling which identified significance. It represents a meta-analysis of seven RCTs related to the effect of steroids on women expected to give birth prematurely. Two of the seven trials showed statistical significance in terms of improving the survival of the child, however the meta-analysis showed that in mothers who received steroids their infants were 30–50 per cent less likely to die.

ACTIVITY

Visit the Cochrane website at www.cochrane.org/ and view the logo

A sensitivity analysis is usually undertaken to identify any changes in the original data that may have occurred as a result of pooling. This involves re-analyzing data from different perspectives to see if this will have an impact on the results. If substantial changes are reported to have occurred as a result of pooling data then caution should be observed in applying the results to your own area of practice.

Meta-synthesis

Meta-synthesis is derived from the Greek words *meta*, meaning 'change, alteration transcend or going beyond', and *synthesis*, meaning 'to put together' (*Collins Dictionary*, 1979), which would suggest this is about putting things together in a way that goes beyond the features of individual items. Finlayson and Dixon (2008) have suggested it is the bringing together of the findings of qualitative research in an effort to provide a clearer picture of the phenomenon of interest. Evans and Pearson (2001) also identified that a meta-synthesis allows for a systematic and critical examination/interpretation.

There are a variety of approaches to meta-analysis, however Pearson et al. (2007) claim that it generally involves:

- data extraction – identifying the research findings in the form of metaphors, themes, categories and/or concepts present within the study;
- data synthesis – grouping the findings into categories;
- grouping the categories into synthesized findings.

The processes involved are very similar to those of primary qualitative research, and as in any form of qualitative research reviewers are providing an interpretation of the findings. The process appears on the face of it to be a simple one, but in reality is quite complex and requires a rigorous examination of studies. The aim is to provide an accurate representation of the findings which gives a full picture of the essential characteristics of the phenomenon under consideration. The specific approach used to achieve this should be clearly outlined to enable you to judge the rigor of the process and the appropriateness of the review for application within your own area of practice.

Whereas heterogeneity is an issue of great concern within meta-analysis, this is less so within meta-synthesis (Evans and Pearson, 2001). In qualitative research heterogeneity is anticipated – the issue for reviewers is to ensure that differences are acknowledged, compared across studies and accounted for within the new interpretation.

Conclusions, recommendations/limitations

Reviewers should justify their conclusions and recommendations in relation both to their application to practice and the implications for health care. Recommendations in terms of future research agendas are normally included. Other information, such as the costs involved in treatment regimes, should also be addressed.

Applicability to practice

The criteria identified in Chapter 5 for judging applicability to practice are equally valid for SRs, however there is also a specific aspect that should be considered. The specificity of the systematic review question means that a very narrow aspect of care is being considered and there is a clear need to place this within the 'bigger picture' of the care environment you are concerned with. You need to consider whether factors not considered in the review will have implications for applying the results to your own area of practice.

EBP ACTIVITY

Identify a systematic review specific to your area of practice and critically appraise it using the criteria identified in Appendix 6.

SUMMARY

- SRs provide a rigorous review of research findings in relation to a specific question and as such they are fundamental to EBP, providing practitioners with sound evidence on which to base practice.
- The SR review process involves the 'pooling' of results from 'like' studies and creating a larger data set for analysis. This is known as meta-analysis in relation to quantitative research and meta-synthesis in relation to qualitative findings.
- If there is significant heterogeneity within studies reviewed in a SR it is unlikely that the results will be subjected to meta-analysis.
- There is a variety of approaches to meta-synthesis, and it is important that a clear description of the approach used is provided to allow you to make decisions as to the rigor of the review.

Further reading

Akobeng, A.K. (2005) 'Understanding systematic reviews and meta-analysis'. Available at: www.adc.bmj.com (accessed August 2008). Gives a good introduction to meta-analysis.

Finlayson, K. and Dixon, A. (2008) 'Qualitative meta-synthesis: A guide for the novice', *Nurse Researcher*, 15 (2): 59–71. Explores the central themes of this approach.

Greenhalgh, T. (2006) *How to Read a Paper: The basics of evidence-based medicine* (3rd edn). Oxford: Blackwell. Provides guidelines for a clear description of how to critique meta-analysis.

E-resources

Campbell Collaboration: prepares, promotes and updates systematic reviews of social interventions.
www.campbellcollaboration.org/MG/index/asp

Centre for reviews and dissemination: has systematic reviews on selected topics, and a database of reviews and resources for the conducting of systematic reviews.
www.york.ac.uk/inst/crd

Cochrane Collaboration: promotes, supports and prepares systematic reviews, mainly in relation to effectiveness.
www.cochrane.org/

Joanna Briggs Institute: promotes evidence-based health care through systematic reviews and a range of resources aimed at promoting evidence synthesis, transfer and utilization.
www.joannabriggs.edu.au

Conclusion to Part 2

The aim of this section was to provide you with the necessary skills, knowledge and tools to enable you to critically appraise a range of evidence. Hopefully you have now:

- identified a number of papers relevant to your own area of practice;
- found a number of appropriate tools to aid you in your critical appraisal;
- identified gaps in your knowledge and developed action plans to allow you to fill in the gaps;
- developed confidence in your ability to critically appraise evidence in an appropriate way.

The section ends with a word search puzzle in which there are 24 words associated with Chapters 5, 6, 7 and 8. What are these? The answers can be found on p. 149.

B	V	O	E	N	K	K	Y	T	I	L	I	B	A	D	N	E	P	E	D
V	D	E	X	Y	C	Z	A	Y	T	I	L	I	B	A	I	L	E	R	O
X	E	T	R	A	I	L	S	E	V	B	N	C	L	O	R	T	N	O	C
S	S	R	Y	T	I	D	I	L	A	V	S	O	N	G	U	W	K	Q	F
I	I	N	I	M	W	E	X	T	G	M	S	M	H	F	Q	W	S	B	L
S	M	K	M	G	Z	D	V	R	E	E	E	F	Q	H	B	I	I	R	S
E	O	L	K	C	O	D	Z	A	N	P	N	I	T	H	W	E	R	A	I
H	D	X	I	I	T	U	A	N	S	W	I	R	M	T	I	G		C	S
T	N	W	S	K	O	N	R	S	T	E	H	M	K	P	P	S	E	K	Y
O	A	A	Y	C	D	C	K	F	R	L	T	A	U	L	R	V	V	E	L
P	R	C	N	R	N	I	T	E	A	B	R	B	Q	L	O	W	I	T	A
Y	O	O	A	E	G	R	P	R	T	A	O	I	Q	A	B	V	T	I	N
H	C	E	E	D	H	T	E	A	I	I	W	L	N	B	A	S	A	N	A
B	O	R	M	I	S	E	O	B	F	R	T	I	L	W	B	D	L	G	
E	F	D	O	B	W	M	G	I	I	A	S	T	K	O	I	E	E	X	A
Y	M	F	T	I	Y	A	A	L	E	V	U	Y	S	N	L	K	R	I	T
M	E	I	E	L	Z	R	W	I	D	O	R	H	L	S	I	K	V	L	E
T	O	C	C	I	V	A	D	T	C	N	T	B	P	K	T	T	Z	S	M
Z	E	D	M	T	Y	P	D	Y	Z	O	F	M	Z	R	Y	G	M	O	P
O	O	X	E	Y	R	E	A	U	R	C	B	V	E	T	I	C	C	F	X

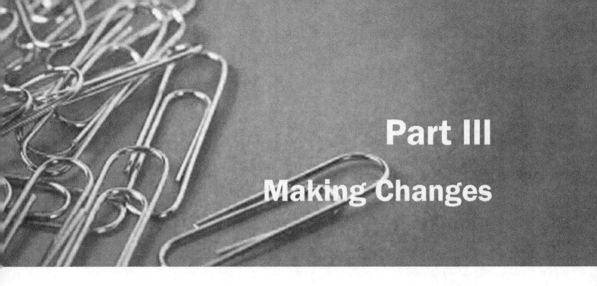

Part III

Making Changes

Moving from Evidence to Practice Development

Introduction

Whilst EBP is generally accepted as a something to aspire to, in reality changes to practices are not easily made. Whilst nurses identify they are confident of their clinical expertise, it has been shown that frequently practice is not based on best evidence. Grol and Grimshaw (2003) found that that between 30 and 40 per cent of patients do not receive care based on sound evidence. The transferring of evidence into practice is often a daunting, difficult and complex activity. Simply informing people of the latest research findings does not mean that new approaches will be adopted and it cannot be assumed that developing people's knowledge and skills will result in practice change – just knowing something does not mean people will choose to do it. For instance, most people know that hand washing is central to reducing infections and yet large numbers of health professionals fail to do this appropriately (see for example Haas and Larson, 2008). Changing care delivery and individuals' behaviours and approaches takes time and effort. It is important to be thoroughly prepared before trying to instigate change. There is no single best way of introducing new evidence into practice, as the type of change required will often dictate the approach to be used. The intention of this chapter is to give you an overview of the issues you need to consider and the tools that may be of use to you.

What does moving from evidence into practice mean?

There are different terms used for putting evidence into practice. Much has been written about **change management**, where various theoretical models outlining the processes and mechanisms that can be used for making changes to behaviours and practices are described. The advent of EBP has brought with it the term 'implementing evidence-based practices', which considers how evidence – and in particular research – can be applied in the practice setting. 'Knowledge translation', 'knowledge/evidence utilization' and 'research implementation' are also used to describe the processes involved in applying knowledge/evidence to a practice setting. Just as there are a plethora of terms there is also a range of approaches and it can seem difficult to navigate your way through these. However, the central premise for all these terms and models is the need to ensure that health professionals' clinical practice is effective and based on sound and current evidence.

Why new knowledge is not incorporated into practice

As highlighted above, much of current practice is not based on sound evidence and yet a great deal of time is dedicated to teaching professionals about the need for evidence-based practice and trying to develop the necessary skills to facilitate this approach. Tingle (2002) investigated newly qualified nurses' experiences of changing practice and found that while individuals were aware of the need to change certain practices in their own working environment, many felt they were not able to do anything about this due to a lack of confidence and experience and also a lack of support from other staff and/or their manager.

ACTIVITY

Consider your own area of practice. Identify those factors which would help and those which would act as barriers to making changes in practice.

MacGuire (1990) has suggested that a number of issues impact on nurses' use of research findings in practice. These relate to a lack of awareness of the latest research, either through too little information – individuals failing to keep up to date – or information overload – too much information to synthesize – or because of a lack of relevant information for their sphere of practice – research not being undertaken. She also suggested a time lag was apparent in relation to the use of relevant evidence. Often practices will be considered safe, having been based on evidence, but frequently this will be out-of-date theory. The time between evidence being generated and practice being adopted in a setting could be huge.

Four main reasons for the under-use of research in practice have been put forward by Rycroft–Malone et al. (2004b):

1. Inability to interpret the research findings.
2. A lack of organizational support.
3. Research seen as lacking clinical credibility.
4. Nurses prefer a clinical specialist to tell them of the latest developments.

Thompson et al. (2008) argued that nurses preferred to rely on experiential sources of knowledge. (The proposed 'top five' sources of information and the least used can be seen in Table 9.1.) Scott et al. (2008) support the idea that nurses rely on this experiential knowledge and clinical expertise gained through their own and others' experiences, and also suggest this type of knowledge is valued because it is specific to the context in which nurses work, as well as readily accessible and patient-centred. Research, on the other hand, tends to be seen as less easy to access, and often not specifically relevant to the sorts of issues nurses are faced with. Nurses also appear to prefer others (such as nurse specialists) to provide them with research evidence rather than seek it out themselves.

Table 9.1   *Sources of information most/least used by nurses*

Top five information sources	Least used sources of information
1. Individual patients and personal experience.	1. Journals.
2. In-service mechanisms.	2. 'Custom and practice'.
3. Nurse education.	3. The media.
4. Discussions with doctors and fellow nurses.	
5. Intuition.	

It has been proposed that in any change required at team level and above, 15 per cent of people involved will be for it, 15 per cent will be against it, and the rest will just go along with any outcome for a quiet life. Some people will also actively sabotage efforts. Often there is what MacGuire (1990) has described as the 'shifting sands syndrome' – at each point of the process of change, barriers are identified by participants to prevent anyone taking the next step ('It can't be done because ...'). Bridges (2003) argued the most difficult part of making a change is getting people to let go of their usual practices. People prefer what is 'familiar' to them and are therefore often resistant to what they see as a threat to their normal activities and likely to increase their stress levels. McPhail (1997) refers to this as 'comfort zones', which nurses develop over time and are reluctant to change unless they become disenchanted with particular established practices. Moving people out of their comfort zone is not an easy task and can be at the heart of whether change is successful or not. Concerns may relate to beliefs (either real or imagined) about what the change will mean for them and can come from:

- fear of the unknown;
- uncertainty about the value of the change;
- a lack of knowledge and/or skills;
- a lack of confidence in the ability to meet new demands;
- feelings of powerlessness;
- resentment if change is seen as unnecessary.

Greenhalgh et al. (2004) identified five key factors associated with a person's willingness to implement changes to practice (see Box 9.1).

Box 9.1   Factors associated with an individual willingness to change

1. Psychological factors – a person's characteristics which may predispose them to innovation of practices, such as a tolerance of ambiguity, intellectual ability, motivation, values and learning style.
2. Context-specific issues – the motivation to make changes and 'fit' with individual needs is likely to make someone implement changes in practice.
3. Meaning – the meaning the change has for an individual is central to whether or not they will choose to make changes to their practice.
4. Nature of the decision – this may depend on other things being in place, such as acceptance by others or being told by others to make a change.
5. Information needs – the meeting of these appropriately throughout the process of change.

It has also been suggested that if change is forced on people they may move into their 'panic zone' and because of the emotions evoked will not be able to make the changes proposed (NHS Institute of Innovation and Improvement, 2005). However, if people are only moved into a 'discomfort zone' through the use of appropriate implementation strategies and are then supported through the process they are more likely to change their practices.

ACTIVITY

Imagine that you have been told you need to change a particular aspect of your practice. What feelings would this evoke and what would be your most likely response?

Two further obstacles to change have been proposed by McPhail (1997) – a lack of shared vision and a lack of forward planning. The lack of a shared vision can lead to a 'them' and 'us' situation, where it is felt that 'they' want 'us' to change for no good reason. This may also be supported by a feeling that the work required is not appreciated by 'them' and all the hard work is left to 'us'. Unless there are sufficient numbers of people committed to a change, who share the same vision, then any attempt to implement this is likely to fail. If people have the skills associated with, and see the benefits to, implementing a new practice they are more likely to be motivated to make a change. Finally, the lack of forward planning is a major barrier to implementing new practices and is discussed in more depth below.

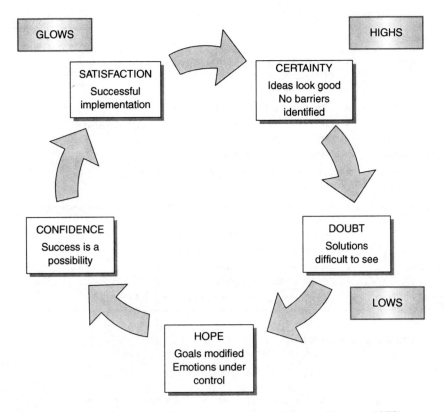

Figure 9.1   *Emotional cycle of change (adapted from Kelley and Connor, 1979)*

Kelley and Connor (1979) have described an 'emotional cycle of change', out-lining the feelings people are likely to experience when going through the change process. As can be seen in Figure 9.1, this is a series of 'highs' and 'lows' that will hopefully culminate in the 'glow' of success. When implementing new practices this must been done at an appropriate pace, thereby giving people enough time to adjust to and think through any proposed changes.

Upton and Brooks (1995) offer a 'change equation' – f(D,V,S) > R. They suggest that successful change will be achieved where:

A combination of the **f**actors

$$\left.\begin{array}{l}\textbf{D}\text{issatisfaction with current practices} \\[1em] \textbf{V}\text{ision for a better future} \\[1em] \textbf{S}\text{teps are planned to achieve goals}\end{array}\right\}$$

**IS
GREATER
THAN**

Resistance
to the
change

As can be seen there are a number of factors that can impact on implementing changes to practice and there is a need to address these before such changes can be made. The characteristics associated with promoting change are summarized in Table 9.2.

Table 9.2   *Elements required to promote change*

Element	Features
Involvement	• All individuals affected by the proposed change – service users, professionals and carers. • Creating ownership.
Motivation	• A valuing and respecting of everyone's contribution.
Planning	• Considering all aspects of the change and potential issues. • Creating a positive environment.
Legitimization	• Owned by all those involved.
Education	• Development of necessary skills or knowledge.
Management	• Appropriate facilitation and guidance.
Expectations	• Having a flexible approach, expecting the unexpected, and respecting others' experiences. • Anticipating conflict and resistance.
Nurturance	• Recognizing the needs of individuals.
Support	• Active listening to concerns. • Providing access to resources.
Trust	• Open, honest and clear communication of information.

Implementing new practice

According to Akerman (1997) there are three types of change:

- developmental – the enhancement or further development of current practices;
- transitional – moving from current practice to other desired ways of working;
- transformational – radical change which significantly alters the structure and processes of an organization.

Shanley (2007) echoed this model, proposing different 'levels of intensity' in relation to changing practice. Change can occur on a personal, team, organizational, national or even global level.

    If you are a student nurse or a newly qualified nurse the thought of making changes to practice beyond a personal level is probably not high on your agenda. In learning to be a nurse, much of your energy must be focused on learning how to do things appropriately. Nevertheless, it is important to remember that what you learn in Year 1 of a pre-registration course may be out of date by the time you are in Year 3. So one of the first priorities in implementing evidence-based practice is to ensure your own practice is based on up-to-date evidence. In making a change at an individual level there is still a need to consider patient preferences identifying whether:

- the change is appropriate to the patients' expressed preferences;
- patients are aware of their options in terms of care delivery and able to make an informed choice;
- it is ethically and culturally acceptable to the patient;
- it is practicable in the context your practice is in;
- you have the knowledge, skills and resources to implement the change.

There is also a need to discuss changes with practice colleagues to ensure that your actions do not cause friction or difficulties within the care team and do not run counter to the care philosophy of your area of practice.

Five 'pearls' are offered by Butz (2007) which can give a starting point for developing EBP and implementing changes into practice at a personal and team level as well as creating an EBP culture:

1. Personal development – making a commitment to accessing databases on a regular basis.
2. Team discussions – timetabling regular meeting with colleagues to discuss ideas and information and to identify areas for change.
3. Culture of inquiry – promoting and developing an inquiry approach in your area of practice.
4. Research relationships – encouraging the development of relationships that may result in research activities.
5. Disseminate evidence – creating systems for sharing information and best practice evidence.

ACTIVITY

Consider the five 'pearls' above. Choose two and identify how you could build these into your work life.

The PARIHS (Promoting Action on Research Implementation in Health Services) framework, developed by a Royal College of Nursing project group (Rycroft-Malone, 2004), draws together three elements that are thought to be central to the success of making changes to practice:

1. Evidence – its clarity.
2. Context – its quality.
3. Facilitation – the type needed.

For change to be successfully brought about it is suggested that the evidence on which changes are to be based needs to be seen as being of good quality, valued and viewed as relevant by both the clinical staff and the patients/service users. Grol and Grimshaw (2003) proposed the characteristics of the evidence can have a major influence on whether that evidence is integrated into practice, and also argued that some evidence will be easier to integrate into practice than others. If evidence reflects widespread concerns in relation to particular practices, or is seen as supporting professional group values, then it is more likely to be adopted. The quality of evidence also impacts on its uptake, for example guidelines that are seen as clear, explicit and straightforward are more likely to be implemented.

The context in which care is delivered is itself seen as constantly changing. Patients come and go, their conditions change or may deteriorate rapidly, and working with other health-care professionals brings with it its own complexities. If change is to be made against this sort of background there is a need for individuals to feel valued, for the necessary resources to be readily available, and for effective teamwork practices.

For change in practice to happen it needs to be facilitated by someone. The type of facilitation and the facilitator are seen as central to this process, which needs to be enabling and empowering and must include all those parties involved in the decision-making process. Change at team level and beyond therefore needs to be facilitated by someone who is prepared to take on the role of **change agent** supported by senior members of staff. Rycroft-Malone's (2002) work suggested this needed to be someone who is part of the team and present in the day-to-day activities, who can see the change as appropriate and can therefore motivate individuals. The characteristics of a good facilitator can be seen in Box 9.2.

Box 9.2   Characteristics associated with a good facilitator

Flexibility	Commitment
Persistence	Presence
Negotiating	Project management
Facilitation	Persuasive
Credibility	Sincerity
Leadership	Clarity of vision
Good communicator	

It has been proposed that the knowledge/skills associated with the change agent role are developed slowly, in a step-by-step and often haphazard way (Greenhalgh, 2006). So if you are participating in facilitating changes to practice beyond those within your personal control, you need to start in a small way and then develop those skills and approaches over time.

The process of implementing evidence-based practice

There are various models available to guide the process of changing practice (see Table 9.3 for examples). These all have certain aspects in common, including the need for planning, implementation and evaluation strategies to be in place. Iles and Sutherland (2001) suggest that it is important that these aspects are not seen as being separate and discrete stages that must be undertaken in isolation. It is likely, no matter how thorough the planning, that issues will arise which have not been considered, therefore planning must remain a continuous process. The implementation phase needs to be evaluated at all stages to ensure that what is intended to happen does indeed do so. As issues arise further planning and then implementation will be needed, with an evaluation of the impact of those adjustments already made. As Schon (1983) describes, there are areas of professional practice where evidence can be easily used to support practice – the high hard ground – however, more frequently practice occurs in 'messy' and 'swampy lowlands' where there are challenging problems which will frequently impact on the rigorous application of evidence to practice.

The planning stage will usually involve what is known as a diagnostic analysis. As Nickols (2000) suggests, change is a problem-solving activity which usually starts with a diagnosis of the problem, allowing the goals to be identified and the

Table 9.3   *Models for promoting change*

Brady and Lewin (2007)	Lewin (1951)	Metz et al. (2007)
1. Plan – involve all affected by the change. Identify outcomes. Pilot proposals. Identify motivators. 2. Implement – establish a realistic time-line with built in evaluation points. 3. Correct – be flexible and address issues as they arise. 4. Communicate – use multiple ways of keeping people informed. 5. Evaluate – identify impact of changes for both professionals and service users.	• Unfreeze – Recognition of the need for change. • Moving – Making the change by altering behaviours or activities. • Refreeze – embedding the change in practice.	1. Exploration – change/ implementation of ideas considered. 2. Preparation – resources needed identified and made available. 3. Early implementation – initial adjustments to implement practices made. 4. Full implementation – all staff have appropriate level of competency and change is fully embedded in their activities. 5. Sustainability – skills, knowledge and resources are maintained at the required level to ensure change remains in place. 6. Innovation – consideration of adaptations and other changes required.

strategies by which these can be achieved put in place. The 'problem' considered in relation to EBP is moving from one practice to another, and therefore the diagnosis analysis will involve a consideration of the area or context within which change is to be made. The idea is to identify any barriers, organisational and/or professional issues which must be taken into account before any attempt is made to implement change. This also allows for the identification of the gap between what is currently happening and what the vision for the future is. Highlighting that gap makes planning the implementation easier and also reduces the likelihood of unforeseen problems and barriers to changing practices.

One of the simplest and easiest approaches to consider the issues around making a change is to use a SWOT analysis – Strengths, Weaknesses, Opportunities, and Threats. An alternative to SWOT is the Seven S model (see Table 9.4).

ACTIVITY

Identify an area of practice that you would like to change and undertake using either a SWOT (a template is provided in appendix 1) or 7S model to identify the issues you would need to consider.

An alternative to the two models above is the 'how, what and why' approach. These question types reflect the various approaches to change that different

Table 9.4   *7S model*

Element	Features
Staff	• What is needed – number, skill mix, characteristics (attitudes, values, etc)?

Skills	• What is needed and what is available in relation to:
	  o clinical/technical skills?
	  o interpersonal skills?
	  o managerial skills?
	  o research/EBP skills?

Structure	• What are the current features of the organization? • What is needed? • What is the 'fit' between the two?
Systems	• Which are present and which are needed?
Strategy	• What is the plan? • What are the priorities?
Style (management)	• What is the current style? • Does this fit with what is needed to achieve the planned changes?
Shared beliefs	• What beliefs and values are present? • Which are needed to achieve the planned change? • Is there a gap between the two?

people will take within organizations – namely, their 'mind set'. Working through these questions can help to address all the issues that need to be considered and planned for:

- How do I get my colleagues to change from X to Y intervention?
- What do I want to achieve, what changes have to be made, and what will indicate success?
- Why is intervention X used and why do we need to change to Y?

ACTIVITY

Consider the SWOT or 7S analysis you undertook in relation to your chosen area of practice. Does the 'how, what, why' approach provide information you hadn't considered previously?

Once all the issues that may impact on implementing change and the resources needed have been identified, planning how to make that change must be undertaken. There is a need here to set realistic goals, to identify a time line and draw up an implementation strategy. Changing practice takes time, and all those who the change will affect should be involved with time to ensure there is adequate consultation and planning.

Implementation has its own specific areas for consideration. Metz et al. (2004) have suggested there are three types of implementation:

1. Paper – where policies are in place but no changes to practice actually occur.
2. Fragmented – where new structures are put in place but are not targeted at the right people: therefore those involved are unable to develop the necessary skills and once again practice remains unchanged.
3. Impact implementation – where strategies and structures are appropriate and are designed specifically to ensure practice change.

As can be seen, not all proposed changes will occur and there are a number of barriers to the successful implementation of change:

- perception of research/evidence – this has to be seen as legitimate;
- staff factors – a lack of experience, knowledge, skills;
- organizational issues – structure, management systems;
- resources – equipment, staff, and so on not available;
- patient/carer perceptions – preference, level of knowledge, availability of information.

In implementing change there is a need to ensure that all these have been taken into consideration and addressed before attempting to make that change. There is also a need to check progress frequently and to ensure feedback is given to people at regular intervals so they are aware of progress and any issues that have arisen. If changes to practice are to be sustained and the practices implemented remain in place, there is a further need to ensure that the necessary resources are maintained and people are rewarded for doing a good job. The NHS Institute of Innovation and Improvement (2007) has suggested that the factors that promote innovation are the same as those that ensure change is sustained. These key factors are identified in Table 9.5.

Table 9.5   *Characteristics associated with sustainability*

Factor	Issues
Practice integration	• Time and resources sufficient to enable integration. • Fits with environment's core beliefs and goals.
Evidence	• Evidence of benefits and effectiveness. • Progress in implementing change.
Readiness	• Staff accept the need for innovation.
Nature of innovation	• Fits with organizational culture. • Where it comes from – top down or bottom up.
Context	• Management style. • Positive environment. • Rewards available.
Engagement	• Staff commitment. • Management of resistance.
Support	• Senior management involvement. • All stakeholders committed to innovation.
Incentives	• Benefits to patients and staff. • Disincentives identified and addressed.

(Continued)

Table 9.5   *(Continued)*

Factor	Issues
Implementation process	• Paced appropriately. • Time-line established. • Good communication.

Resources	• Sufficient, appropriate and ongoing:
	  o staff;
	  o funding;
	  o equipment;
	  o education.

Leadership	• Credible, appropriate and empowering.
'Influencers'	• Champions at all levels in all staff groups.
Relationships	• Effective multi-professional teams. • Common goals. • Roles and responsibilities clearly defined.
Ownership	• All feel involved and part of the process. • Fits specific local needs.

Once a change has been fully integrated into practice there is a need to formally evaluate the implementation of the practice, identifying whether that change has had an appropriate impact on care and the lessons learnt and whether any further innovations are needed. You must be able to see whether or not you have actually arrived at the point you intended and whether the planned change is an improvement on previous practice. Without this evaluation you could end up with a situation where the 'implementation of the change is a success but unfortunately the patient died'. As identified in Chapter 1, evaluation is different to research and audit and has different goals. Evaluation needs to be planned as part of the process of introducing new practices and taking decisions in the planning phase as to what is intended to be evaluated – the effectiveness of the practice, the processes used, the impact of the changes, or all three.

EBP ACTIVITY

Consider the diagnosis analysis you undertook earlier in the chapter and create a possible implementation and evaluation strategy that would enable you to change an aspect of your practice. Discuss the feasibility of your plan with a colleague/peer.

SUMMARY

- Transferring evidence into practice is a complex activity which takes time and effort.
- Comfort zones develop over time and change is unlikely unless nurses are motivated to alter their established practices.

- A shared vision is necessary if change is to be successful and people need to have the skills and to see the benefits of implementing new practice.
- Change can occur on a personal, team, organizational, national or even a global level.
- Strategies and structures need to be designed specifically to ensure practice changes are sustained.

Further reading

Bridges, W. (2003) *Making Transitions: Making the most of change*. London: Nicholas Brealey. A good overview of the principles of making changes to practice.

Metz, A.J.R. Blasé, K. and Bowie, L. (2007) 'Implementing evidence-based practices: six drivers of success. Brief Research-to-Results', *Child Trends*, October. Available at: www.childtrends.org. Provides a step-by-step approach to moving evidence into practice.

Rycroft-Malone, J. (2004) 'The PARIHS Framework – A framework for guiding the implementation of evidence-based practice', *Journal of Nursing Care Quality*, 19 (4): 297–304. Provides a detailed account of the issues to be considered when making changes to practices.

E-resources

National Institute Service Delivery and Organisation Programme: established in 1999 to develop an organization, management and service delivery evidence base, their 'Managing Change' web-page contains various useful documents. http://www.sdo.nihr.ac.uk/managing change.html

The NHS Institution for Innovation and Improvement: provides a series of Improvement Leader guides aimed at providing people with the skills and knowledge to promote service improvement and innovation. www.institute.nhs.uk/products/improvementleadersguidebox set.htm

Reflection, Portfolios and Evidence-Based Practice

Learning Outcomes

By the end of the chapter you will be able to:

- identify the key aspects of lifelong learning;
- apply reflection as an aspect of EBP;
- use reflective approaches to practice;
- discuss your personal and professional development needs;
- identify the key elements of portfolio development.

Introduction

Evidence-based practice is viewed as not only encompassing the use of appropriate research and literature but also embracing lifelong learning as a way to ensure practice is evidence-based. **Lifelong learning** is seen as essential if practitioners are to be able to meet the ever-changing demands of practice. EBP requires that health professionals' knowledge and skills development keeps pace with their practice and evidence development. There is, therefore, a need to develop those skills associated with lifelong learning. **Reflection** and portfolio development are central to this process, as they can enable you to identify your learning needs, set goals for that learning and evaluate whether these have been met appropriately. As a nurse there is a need to be open to learning and the possibility of change, which requires you to continually assess your knowledge and skills and any areas requiring development. This chapter will help you to consider how you can develop the skills of lifelong learning and reflection and ensure your personal and professional development.

Lifelong learning

The idea of lifelong learning comes from general education, appearing in the literature in the early 1970s. It was adopted by nursing with the development of the Post Registration Education and Practice (PREP) requirements imposed by the then nursing regulatory body the UKCC (1995). The importance of lifelong learning was emphasized as a response to the expanding role of nurses and the fast pace of change evident in health-care settings. The NMC (2002) stated that the principles of lifelong learning were 'increasingly important to all registered practitioners' and required all nurses to develop their knowledge and skills, demonstrating this through a portfolio of learning and facilitating by engaging in clinical supervision.

Claxton (1999) described lifelong learning as the ability to identify:

- your learning needs;
- the goals and resources needed to achieve them;
- your strengths and weaknesses;
- your blind spots, inherent assumptions and behaviours;
- your mechanisms for monitoring progress and motivating yourself when you become 'stuck'.

He suggested that it requires 'resilience, resourcefulness and reflection'.

There are two main ways of learning: mediated – aided by a 'teacher' – and unmediated – through experience. Kolb (1984) proposed that learning from experience is a cyclic process whereby experiences are analyzed through the use of reflection to promote learning and generate new ways of working. The four stages are experience; reflective observation; making sense of the experience; and testing new learning. Boud et al. (1985) suggested that people were often unaware of their learning processes, that reflection makes these processes accessible and enabled people to use them more effectively and therefore enhance their lifelong learning.

Leaving learning to 'chance experiences' in relation to EBP is not appropriate and a more structured approach which promotes focused experiential learning through the use of self-direction is needed. Self-directed approaches come from theories of andragogy (how adults learn) and are implicit within lifelong learning. It is suggested that adults are self-directive in their learning, namely that they have a readiness for and a motivation to learn, drawing on their past experience as a resource for learning.

Self-directed learning involves developing the ability to identify what you need to know and how to go about learning it. Knowles (1990) defined four key factors that should be considered when identifying learning needs:

1. Assessment of needs – reflecting on your experiences to identify where you are, where you want to be and what the gap is between the two.
2. Identifying your learning goals.
3. Planning how to meet those goals.
4. Evaluating the outcomes.

Reflective practice

There are many definitions of reflection, however it can basically be said to be the process by which someone actively considers an experience, critically appraising it in light of experience and knowledge and developing a new perspective to be tested in new situations. Therefore reflective practice can be seen as a three-stage cycle (Jasper, 2003):

1. Experience.
2. Critical appraisal.
3. New perspectives.

Williams (2001) put forward three types of reflection:

1. Content – related to the description of an issue by asking 'what' questions (e.g., what happened?).
2. Process reflection – related to asking 'how' questions (e.g., how did it happen?).
3. Premise or critical reflection – related to exploring the why of things (e.g., why were certain judgments made?).

Reflection provides a structure by which to consider experiences. It also helps in considering 'normal' situations in a different way rather than passively accepting practices as appropriate. Reflection is not something that is built into some people's ways of thinking and not others; it can be learnt and developed over time.

Jarvis (1992) suggested that reflective practice requires professionals to look at all practice as a potential learning experience by which they can ensure their personal and professional development. Critical reflection takes this process one step further by encouraging the individual to identify the differences between their actual practice and what is desirable. Reflection can be seen as a form of self-consciousness, whereas critical reflection is about continual self-critique. This is not an easy thing to do but if it is done well it can provide many benefits. Reflection is seen as helping to:

- bridge the theory/practice gap;
- reduce practices based on custom and practice;
- develop an understanding of your practice, the decisions made, the lessons learnt and the implications of these for future practice;
- ensure that care remains patient-centred and based on patient experience.

Schon (1983) identified knowledge as occurring in the form of either technical rationality (knowing facts) or professional artistry (intuitive knowledge), and both are needed if you are to practise effectively as these can be brought together through reflective processes. Critical reflection can provide the opportunity to learn from an experience – what is known as transformational learning – and to adapt practice rather than endlessly repeat the same activity. There are various models available (see Table 10.1 for example) and different ways of undertaking reflection (see Table 10.2 for example). Whilst these all share the same basic element, the best way to approach reflection is to find a way that suits your style of thinking and working.

Schon (1983) suggested that reflection should be undertaken in two ways:

1. Reflecting-in-action – whilst undertaking activities, during the experience of practice. This is the ability to 'think on one's feet' and apply knowledge and past experience to a current situation.
2. Reflecting-on-action – a conscious attempt to reflect after an event.

Table 10.1   *Examples of reflective models*

Gibbs's (1988) reflective cycle	Boud et al. (1985)	John (2006)	Borton (1970)

1. Description – what happened
2. Feelings – what you thought and felt
3. Evaluation – what was good/bad about the experience
4. Analysis – making sense of the events
5. Discussion – what else could have been done
6. Action Plan – what to do now
	1. Experience
	  a. behaviour
	  b. ideas
	  c. feelings
	2. Reflection
	  a. consider
	  b. evaluate
	3. Outcomes
	  a. new perspectives
	  b. changes in behaviour
		1. Description of experience – what is significant
		2. Feelings – own and others
		3. Goals – what I was trying to achieve
		4. Influencing factors – what influenced the way I felt, thought, responded (social, cultural, organizational, cognitive, professional)
		5. Theoretical framework – what theory did or should have informed my actions
		6. Ethical aspects – did I act for the best?
		7. Previous experience – how this linked with my previous experiences
		8. Looking forward – how I might do it differently
		9. Framing – what I have learnt
			1. What? – is the issue/problem? Asking questions such as what happened, what was I doing?
			2. So what? – does this tell/teach/ mean? Asking questions such as so what more do I need to know, so what was I thinking/ feeling, so what could I have done differently?
			3. Now what? – Asking questions such as what do I need to do next time?

He also identified what he called espoused theory and theory-in-use. Espoused theory is knowledge that is said to underpin practice and is generally accepted as the appropriate body of formal knowledge on which to base that practice. Theory-in-use represents the theories actually used when practising – the beliefs, values and thoughts that direct your behaviour. Sometimes the two can be very different. For example, if asked about promoting patient dignity a nurse may advocate the need to ensure privacy, to show respect for individual wishes and to communicate appropriately with an individual, but in performing a task related to personal hygiene may ignore specific patient preference in relation to religious requirements and so on. Reflection can help in uncovering these discrepancies between espoused theory and theory-in-action and also enable you to examine your own biases and personal perspectives.

Table 10.2   *Different styles of reflection*

Method	Types
Individual	Reflective frameworks Critical incident analysis
Facilitated	Guided reflection Peer reflection
Group	Action learning sets
Clinical Supervision	• Individual
	• Pairs
	• Group

ACTIVITY

Consider a recent practice experience and reflect on your actions. Identify what theory was available to underpin your action and what theory you were actually drawing on. Is there a difference between the two and if so why might this be?

As identified in Table 10.2, reflection can either be unsupervised or supervised. Unsupervized reflection is easier to organize and can be done to fit in with your own needs and timetable. In many ways it is less threatening as there are no concerns about what someone may think about what you have done. However, it does mean that there is also no one to challenge your assumption or work through difficult issues with. Supervized reflection is more difficult to organize and more challenging, but does provide an opportunity to share experiences and draw on someone else's experience and expertise. Duffy (2008) has argued that there are '4Rs' to consider in relation to facilitated reflection:

1. Getting the **R**ight facilitator.
2. Choosing the appropriate **R**eflective framework.
3. **R**eadiness to take part in the process.
4. **R**eflecting on the process.

ACTIVITY

Consider what characteristics you would associate with the 'right' facilitator and for what reasons.

Peer feedback is suggested as a way of aiding the reflective process. Here a trusted and valued peer is asked to give constructive feedback in relation to a particular activity or experience. In receiving this 'feedback' another dimension to your activities and an alternative view as to what happened are provided. However, for this to be effective it must be structured and so each party has to be willing to be open and honest with each other.

Reflection can also be undertaken in relation to a range of experiences. Often it will be incidents seen as 'significant' – either because something didn't go as well as anticipated or because something unexpected happened – that are most likely to prompt consideration. However, it is also important to reflect on normal, day-to-day events as these are the ones where practice becomes 'ritualized' and likely to be based on out-of-date evidence.

Reflective writing/journals

Reflection can be undertaken by thinking through things in a structured way, however writing reflectively can add another dimension to the process. There is something about taking thoughts and reproducing them on paper that provides greater clarity and insight into an experience. It supplies a way of ordering your thoughts and freely expressing your feelings and concerns. It also helps to structure your experience and to make links between various ideas and concepts. You can consider issues in a more objective way, returning to the account of your practice at a later date if necessary without having to rely on being able to fully recall all the details. If you reflect regularly – in a reflective diary for instance – it can provide a log of your activities and allow you to consider if there are any recurrent issues that need to be considered in more depth.

Reflective writing should be a creative process that allows for a full expression of your thoughts and feelings, enabling you to explore and clarify the issues surrounding your experience. One of the barriers to reflecting writing is that often writing is seen as part of a specific process (education programmes, practice reports, nursing notes) and therefore people will learn to write in a way that is demanded by others (teachers, mentors, managers). However, this form of writing is aimed at meeting your needs and you need to find a way of doing this that you feel comfortable with. As with all reflection it needs to be structured if it is to aid your learning so you need to find a model that will help you to do this. Box 10.1 provides a framework that may be helpful in your writing. Like all other skills you need to practise this regularly to feel confident in doing it. It is useful to identify specific times when you can reflect and if you are able to make it part of your routine this will become an essential component of your practice.

Box 10.1   Template for reflection

1. Describe a practice experience, writing a concise account of what you did.
2. How did you feel at the time?
3. What knowledge/evidence did you draw on when undertaking the activity?
4. What sources of evidence are you aware of that could support your practice?
5. Is there a need to consider other forms of knowledge/evidence?
6. What are your learning needs?

(Continued)

(Continued)

7. What sources of information/support could you access to help with your learning?
8. How will you meet your learning needs?
9. What does this mean in relation to your future practice?

Clinical supervision

Clinical supervision first appeared in nursing some eighteen years ago, being proposed as a way of helping nurses to cope with the demands of health-care delivery. It gained momentum as it became seen as a way of facilitating aspects of government initiatives in relation to clinical governance, encouraging continuing professional development and improvement through a formal process of professional support. It has also been endorsed by the NMC as a way of improving standards of care and is intended to be a career-long undertaking.

Butterworth et al. (1998: 12) defined it as 'an exchange between professionals to enable the development of professional skills'. Clinical supervision is undertaken between two or more people, with one person identified as the clinical supervisor. Usually the clinical supervisor will have undergone some form of training to prepare for their role. The aim of the supervision is to discuss and explore an aspect of practice or a particular issue in depth in an attempt to understand what has happened and if different approaches are feasible/possible/available in a safe and supportive environment. There are various models available, however the most commonly used are:

*   educative (formative approaches) – aimed at developing a better understanding of individuals' skills/actions and the patient experience;
*   supportive (restorative approaches) – considers emotional responses and the experience of delivering care;
*   managerial (normative approaches) – explores quality issues and ensuring appropriate standards of care.

All these approaches usually involve agreeing a contract that stipulates the format's length and the timing of meetings, confidentiality and the recording of discussions. Many NHS Trusts will have policies in place identifying their expectation of staff in relation to clinical supervision and the form it will take.

Reflection and EBP

Reflection is central to all aspects of EBP, from identifying that there is an issue of concern to implementing changes to practice. Mantzoukas (2007) stated that reflection enables us to unlock the unconscious knowledge on which we base practice, bringing this into our consciousness and thereby allowing our decision-making process to become clearer. It also enables you to link the knowledge gained through experience with more formal types of knowledge and to then identify areas of concern. Reflection as identified in Chapter 3 is an implicit part of clinical

Table 10.3   *Reflection and management of change model*

Stage	Features
Self-observation	• What does the practice involve?
Self-appreciation	• What are my feelings, beliefs, values in relation to the practice?
Self-analysis	• What is the espoused theory to support practice? • What is the theory in action? • Is there a gap between the two?
Self-contemplation	• What is my experience of this practice? • How do I react when performing this activity? • What concepts underpin my practice?
Self-conceptualization	• How do the concepts identified above relate to current evidence related to the practice? • Is there a need to change my practice?
Self-management of change	• What needs to be in place to make the change?
Self-implementation	• What strategies will I use to implement a change to my practice?

decision-making and central to implementing changes to practice. Table 10.3 provides a reflective framework to enhance any consideration of EBP issues and is adapted from Ochieng's (2005) model of reflection.

Page and Meerabeau (2000) suggested that reflection could lead to constructive action in relation to the planning, implementation and evaluation of change. However, there needs to be a clear link between reflection and actions – making changes to one's own behaviour will not come about without a clear and proactive action plan and the motivation to put that plan into action.

'Doing reflection'

In reflection there is no 'one-size-fits-all' approach and you will need to consider what will work best for you. There are, however, a few basic things that you need to implement in order to be successful.

- experiment with different approaches until you find one that 'fits';
- commit to giving time to reflection in whatever form you choose. See it as an essential aspect to your practice rather than an 'add on';
- start small and work up to the big issues;
- be open to new ideas and new ways of thinking;
- be willing to challenge your assumptions and practices.

ACTIVITY

Consider your own needs in relation to reflection and create an action plan to structure your learning in this area using the above steps to guide you.

Portfolios

Portfolios have been around for a number of years and have been particularly embraced by nurse education. Various definitions are available: McMullan et al. (2003: 289), for example, defined portfolios as 'a collection of evidence, usually in written form, of both the products and processes of learning. It attests to achievements and personal and professional development, by providing critical analysis of its contents'. Alternatively Brown (1992) proposed it was 'a private collection of evidence which demonstrates the continuing acquisition of skills, knowledge, attitudes and activity of the individual'. All definitions have the same themes running through them – that portfolios are a collection of evidence that can provide a picture of your personal and professional development.

There are four main reasons for producing a portfolio:

* learning and development – to demonstrate progress over time;
* professional development – to meet statutory requirements to demonstrate you have kept up to date (e.g., for the NMC);
* assessment – as part of a course to enable an assessment of learning;
* presentation – to showcase your achievements, for example at an interview.

Portfolios are seen as a way of actively engaging people in their own learning, providing a vehicle through which to explore the process and provide evidence of learning.

Portfolios also promote self-directed learning and development, requiring you as a learner to take control of and responsibility for your own learning. In turn they provide a framework for reflecting on your personal and professional development. Most nurses will have had experience of keeping a portfolio as part of their formal education – if you are a pre-registration student or a newly qualified nurse you will no doubt have been required to keep one in some shape or form. The advent of the Agenda for Change career structure (DoH, 2006) and the identification of the Knowledge Skills Framework both indicated that a portfolio of some kind is needed to demonstrate learning and the meeting of agreed developmental goals for registered nurses. Using this to direct your own learning in relation to EBP can seem a daunting task. However, there are key issues that can be adopted to direct your activities: a possible framework is proposed below.

1. Reflect on a practice issue to provide a view of where you are and where you want to be and therefore your learning needs.
2. Identify the learning goals to be achieved by using frameworks such as SMART (see Box 10.2).
3. Undertake a SWOT analysis to enable you to identify which issues are likely to impact on your ability meet your goals (see the template in Appendix 1), enabling you to generate an action plan (see the template in Appendix 7) to achieve your goals.
4. Implement the action plan to collect 'evidence' of your learning.

5. Evaluate your progress and adapt your plan as you develop.
6. On meeting your goal/s the process can begin again.

If the above steps are followed and the documentation is completed this will provide you with a portfolio for your development and learning over time and enable you to both monitor and provide evidence of your progress.

Box 10.2   Setting goals using SMART

In setting goals there is a need to ensure that these are clear and specific. Using the SMART Framework will enable you to achieve this:

Specific – clearly written.
Measurable – written in behavioural terms showing what will be evident when you have achieved your goal so you will know when you have done so.
Achievable – something within your reach.
Relevant – to your context and development needs.
Time limited – clearly identify the time period within which you will meet the goal.

So a goal after using SMART might look something like:

Identify if there are clinical guidelines in relation to practice X in context Y using EBP search engine A and the CINHAL database by (date in two weeks' time).

Personal development planning

Personal development planning is viewed as a structured approach by which individuals can reflect on their current knowledge, skills and achievement, and plan their personal and professional development needs. Mulhall and Le May (2001) proposed that to make the transition to EBP there is a need for individual nurses to actively plan their own personal and professional development to ensure that they already have and can maintain the necessary skills and knowledge associated with their area of practice. This includes thinking about your developmental needs in terms of further study and experience. A template for a personal development plan is provided in Appendix 8 and it may be worth considering what your education and training needs are to ensure you have the skills and knowledge to be an effective practitioner capable of EBP.

EBP ACTIVITY

Identify an area of practice and using the above framework and tools create an action plan for developing your learning in this area.

SUMMARY

- Lifelong learning, reflection and portfolio development are central aspects of EBP.
- People are often unaware of their learning processes and reflection makes these processes accessible and enables people to use them more effectively.
- Self-directed learning involves identifying what you need to know and how to go about learning this.
- Reflective practice has three elements – experience, reflection, and action – and thus provides a structure through which to consider experiences.
- There are three approaches to clinical supervision – educative, supportive, and managerial.
- Portfolios provide a framework through which to structure learning.
- Personal development planning is a structured approach to reflect on current knowledge, skills and achievement, and plan personal and professional development needs.

Further reading

Bond, M. and Holland, S. (1998) *Skills of Clinical Supervision for Nurses*. Buckingham: Open University Press. A good introduction to clinical supervision.

Jasper, M. (2003) *Beginning Reflective Practice*. Cheltenham: Nelson Thornes. Gives a clear overview of various aspects of reflection.

Rolfe, G., Freshwater, D. and Jasper, M. (2001) *Critical Reflection for Nursing and the Helping Professions: A Users Guide*. Hampshire: Palgrave. A good introduction to reflection and the use of clinical supervision.

Timmins, F. (2008) *Making Sense of Portfolios: A guide for nursing students*. Berkshire: Open University Press. Provides a good introduction to portfolios and their uses.

Conclusion to Part 3

The aim of this section was to provide you with the necessary skills, knowledge and tools to enable you to make changes to your practice as appropriate and ensure your practice continues to be an evidence base throughout your career. Hopefully you will have now:

1. Identified ways in which changes can be made to practice and any issues you need to consider before making changes.
2. Considered how best to reflect on your experiences and use that reflection to enhance your practice.
3. Identified your needs in relation to lifelong learning.
4. Developed confiedence in your ability to use evidence appropriately in the delivery of care.

This section ends with a crossword puzzle, with answers to the clues relevant to Chapters 9 and 10. The answers can be found on page 150.

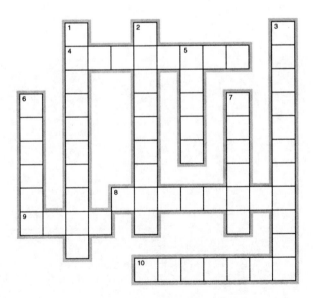

Across

4. theory said to underpin practice
8. learning aimed at ensuring knowledge/skills are up to date
9. a form of analysis that allows you to identify areas for personal development
10. zone where people prefer to practice

Down

1. active appraisal of actions in a structured and critical way
2. a collection of evidence demonstrating learning and development
3. someone who facilitates changes in practice
5. framework for defining goals
6. RCN framework for considering implementation of change
7. plan identifying how needs are met

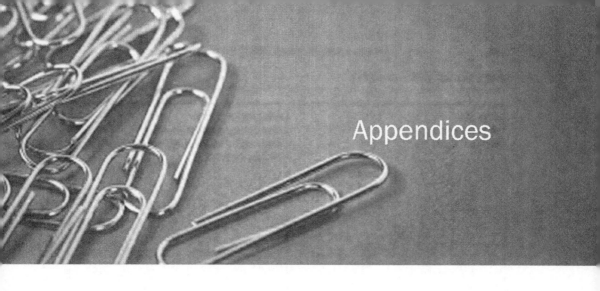

Appendices

Appendix 1: SWOT analysis

Strengths What are my strengths? What am I good at?	Weaknesses What are my current limitations? What might I do/think that would stop me meeting my goal?
Opportunities What will help in achieving my goal? What resources are available to me?	Threats What barriers are there to achieving my goal, both personal and organizational?

Appendix 2: Template for description of EBP interventions

Name of intervention:	
Description (mode of delivery, frequency, restriction):	
Extent of effectiveness:	
Goal to be achieved:	
What will be required of the patient?	
Benefits:	
Risks:	
Side effects:	

Appendix 3: General critical appraisal tool research studies

Section	Things to consider
Title	• Does it clearly identify the area of study?
Abstract	• Does it contain enough information for you to decide whether or not the paper is of interest to you?
Author qualifications	• Are these appropriate for the area of study?
Introduction	• Does it clearly outline the area of interest and give a rationale for the paper? • Is the research question and/or hypothesis clearly identified? • Is a theoretical/conceptual framework identified?
Literature review	• Is there a critical review of the literature related to the area of study? • Is the literature appropriate, up to date, mainly from primary sources, and does it include any seminal works associated with the topic?
Conceptual/ theoretical framework	• Are concepts clearly defined? • Is there a fit between the conceptual framework and the research design?
Ethical issues	• Has ethical approval been acquired? • Are the potential risks and benefits discussed? • Are sources of funding and outside interests identified?
Design	• Is the design clearly stated/described, allowing for its replication? • Is it appropriate to the study? • Are the strengths and limitations debated?
Methodology	• Is this appropriate to the research question/hypothesis and aims of the study? • How are the data to be collected? • What sampling methods are used and are these appropriate to the methodology? • Are issues of reliability, validity, trustworthiness and rigor considered?
Results	• Does it give a clear description of how the results were reached? • Are the results clearly described and presented in a way that promotes understanding?
Discussion	• Are all the results explored and explained? • Is there consistency between the results and the arguments put forward? • Are the arguments logically developed and taking account of opposing views? • Is the interpretation offered reasonable and does it make sense in light of what you know about the subject area?
Conclusions	• Are these logical and coherent? • Do these 'fit' with the data and the arguments presented in the discussion?
Recommendation/ Limitations	• Are these presented in a clear way? • Is there a logical link between the findings and the recommendations?
Applicability to practice	• Is the sample used similar to the patients/service users in your area of practice? • Is training required to implement these findings? • Are considerations such as cost accounted for? • Do the benefits of changing practice outweigh any harmful effects identified?

Appendix 4: Critical appraisal tool for quantitative research studies

Area	Issues for consideration
Hypothesis/research question	• Are the research questions and/or hypothesis clear, unambiguous and where appropriate capable of being tested? • Are these consistent with the conceptual framework and research design?
Literature review	• Is there a critical review of the literature related to the area of study? • Is the literature appropriate, up to date, mainly from primary sources, and does it include any seminal works associated with the topic?
Conceptual/theoretical framework	• Are concepts clearly defined? • Is there a fit between the conceptual framework and the research design?
Operational definitions	• Are all terms used clearly defined? • Do these identify how variables will be observed and measured?
Design	• Is the design clearly stated/described, allowing for its replication? • Is it appropriate to the study? • Are issues which may result in bias minimized? • Are the strengths and limitations debated?
Data collection methods	• Are these adequately described? • Are the instruments adequately described and appropriate to the study's purpose and design? • Are the instruments used valid, reliable and reproducible?
Sampling method	• Is the population of interest identified? • Are the subject characteristics clearly identified? • Are the inclusion and exclusion criteria clearly identified and appropriate? • Is the sampling approach appropriate to the design? • Is the size of sample identified and adequate? • Are power calculations present where appropriate?
Ethical issues	• Has ethical approval been acquired? • Are the potential risks and benefits discussed? • Are sources of funding and outside interests identified?
Data analysis	• Is it appropriate to the type of data? • Is complete information reported? • Is there an adequate description of any subjects who were withdrawn from the study?
Findings	• Are these presented in a clear and understandable way? • Do the tables/charts make sense? • Are data described in sufficient detail?
Discussion	• Is it balanced, including all the major findings? • Are the results considered in light of other research? • Does it address issues of generalizability? • Is there an acknowledgement of limitations?
Validity, reliability, applicability	• Are the results valid and reliable? • Is the relevance for practice identified?

Appendix 5: Critical appraisal tool for qualitative research

Area	Issues for consideration
Research question and aims	• Is the question clearly stated and appropriate to the topic area? • Are the aims clearly stated and relevant to the research question?
Literature review	• Is there a critical review of the literature related to the area of study? • Is the literature appropriate, up to date, mainly from primary sources, and does it include any seminal works associated with the topic?
Conceptual/ theoretical framework	• Are concepts clearly defined? • Is there a fit between the conceptual framework and the research design?
Design	• Is the design clearly stated/described allowing for its replication? • Is it appropriate to the study? • Are the strengths and limitations debated?
Methodology	• Is a qualitative approach appropriate? • Is a specific approach used and described? • Does the research give a clear justification for the research design?
Reflexivity	• Does the researcher(s) provide a statement identifying their position/perspective?
Ethical issues	• Has ethical approval been acquired? • Are the potential risks and benefits discussed? • Are sources of funding and outside interests identified?
Sampling/ participants	• Is the sampling method appropriate and clearly described?
Data collection	• Are the data collection methods appropriate to the research approach and design? • Are the methods described in enough detail for you to understand the process?
Data analysis	• Is the data analysis tool identified and appropriate to the type of data and research design?
Findings	• Are the findings presented in a clear way? • Is there sufficient information to understand how the findings were reached? • Are the findings credible? • Are these discussed in light of other research/literature? • Are the study's limitations identified?
Conclusions	• Are these logical and coherent? • Do these 'fit' with the data and arguments presented in the discussion?
Issues of rigor	• Have steps been taken to ensure the findings have credibility, transferability, dependability, confirmability and authenticity?
Applicability to practice	• Is the sample used similar to the patients/service users in your area of practice? • Is training required to implement the findings? • Are considerations such as cost accounted for? • Do the benefits of changing practice outweigh any harmful effects identified?

Appendix 6: Critical appraisal tool for systematic reviews

Area	Issues for consideration
Question	• Is there a clear and precisely defined question? • Are all terms/concepts clearly and operationally defined? • Are the inclusion and exclusion criteria clearly identified?
Search strategy	• What terms are identified to locate studies and are these appropriate/exhaustive? • What databases were accessed and were these appropriate? • Was a thorough search of all literature sources undertaken?
Quality appraisal	• How was the quality of the studies assessed? • Is there a checklist identified for critical appraisal? • Did two or more people appraise the literature? • Did appraisers provide a rationale for the exclusion of any study?
Data extraction	• Is there evidence that adequate information about sample characteristics was extracted? • Is there sufficient information about the findings extracted?
Summarizing the evidence	• Where meta–analysis/synthesis is not used is this adequately justified? • Are the methods of 'pooling' data clearly explained?
Meta-analysis	• Is the data analysis thorough and credible? • Are treatment effects reported for all relevant outcomes? • How large is the treatment effect?
Meta-synthesis	• Is the heterogeneity of treatment effects adequately addressed? • Were two or more people involved in the data extraction, ensuring the integrity of the dataset? • Is a fuller understanding of the phenomenon of interest achieved? • Are the interpretations appropriate and sound? • Are examples of data provided to support the interpretations? • Were two or more people involved in the data extraction, ensuring the integrity of the dataset?
Conclusions	• Are these coherent and do they flow on naturally from the findings? • Is the strength of the evidence discussed?
Recommendations/ limitations	• What recommendations are made? • Are any potential limitations identified?
Applicability to practice	• Are the implications for practice explored? • How similar is the population of the studies to the patient group I am interested in?

Appendix 7: Action planning

Goal: What do I want to achieve?

Rationale: Why?

Action: How will I go about it?

Criteria for success: How will I know when I've got there?

Evaluation: What have I achieved and what next?

Appendix 8: Personal development plan

What do I want to achieve (goals)?	How will this help my personal development?	How will I achieve this?	What help do I need?
1.			
2.			
3.			

Evaluation:

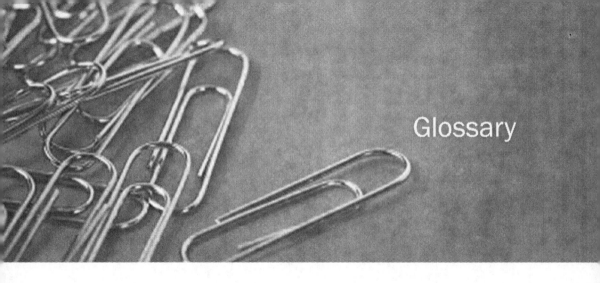

A priori: knowledge arrived at through reasoning processes

Authority: knowledge coming from a source or person viewed as being authoritative

Background question: generally a broad who, what, where, when, how, why question about an area of clinical interest

Bracketing: a process used in qualitative research, where own thoughts and feelings in relation to the study are acknowledged and then 'placed on one side' to allow an unbiased analysis of the data

Care bundles: three or five items of practice evidence grouped together in relation to a particular condition, treatment and/or procedure which have a more positive impact on treatment outcomes than any one element

Change agent: someone who facilitates change in the practice setting by using specific interventions to implement, and evaluate evidence-based practice

Change management: the process of promoting change through the use of specific management theories and approaches

Citation Pearl Growing: a way of identifying literature of interest by using an initial article (pearl) of interest to identify appropriate subject headings

Clinical audit: an approach whereby clinical practices are measured against agreed explicit standards to promote clinical effectiveness

Clinical effectiveness: the delivery of care in the most appropriate and evidence-based way

Clinical governance: the process and structures put in place within health-care institutions to promote and maintain the quality of care

Confirmability: the process of creating an audit trail of decisions taken in relation to the analysis of qualitative data

Correlation study: quantitative research approach which examines relationships between variables without manipulation of the independent variable

Credibility: processes put in place to ensure the findings of qualitative research are seen to be appropriate and representing the participants' experiences

Critical appraisal: a careful evaluation of the worth, value or quality of evidence

Cross-sectional studies: research which compares different groups within a population of interest, collecting data at a single identified point in time

Data saturation: a term used in grounded theory research to indicate the point where no new information is being generated during the collection of data through the use of interviews

Deductive reasoning: reasoning which moves from general theories to a specific hypothesis

Dependability: a term used for assessing the quality of qualitative research by identifying the need to ensure all participant perspectives are accounted for in the analysis of data and the presentation of findings

Descriptive studies: quantitative research which observes, describes, and documents areas of interest as they occur naturally

Disproportional sampling: a form of sampling used in quantitative research where a larger sample of a particular subgroup (e.g., age, ethnicity, etc) is present within a population and usually used where there is a need to consider the relationship between variables in that group

Emic perspective: from the individual's rather than an outsider's or researcher's perspective

Empiricism: a belief that only that which can be observed can be called a fact or truth

Etic perspective: outsider or researcher perspective, rather than a research participant perspective

Evidence: an organized body of knowledge used to support or justify actions and beliefs

Evidence-based medicine: an approach to the delivery of medical practice aimed at ensuring all activities are based on rigorous evidence

Foreground question: a focused question formed in relation to a specific issue and looking for particular knowledge

Gateway site: an electronic device which provides access to specific resources, databases and publications

Grey literature: literature which has not been formally published, including theses and/or dissertations, conference proceedings, and in-house publications, such as leaflets, newsletters, and pamphlets

Hermeneutics: related to meaning and interpretation – how people interpret their experiences within a specific context

Hypothesis: a simple statement identifying a testable relationship between at least two clearly stated variables

Inductive reasoning: reasoning which flows from thoughts related to a particular issue to a general theory

Interpretivism: an alternative to positivism based on the belief that humans are actively involved in constructing their understanding of the world

Intuitive knowledge: a form of tacit knowledge which involves arriving at conclusions without being aware of thinking in a rational and logical way to generate that knowledge

Lifelong learning: self-directed learning in which the aim is to ensure that one's knowledge and skills remain up to date

Longitudinal studies: research in which data are collected at various points over an extended period of time from an identified individual/group of people

MeSH terms: medical subject headings commonly used in certain databases to describe the contents of an article

Meta-analysis: the pooling of data from a number of quantitative research studies to provide a larger dataset

Meta-synthesis: the pooling of findings from a number of qualitative research studies

Paradigm: a collection of ideas and concepts providing a theoretical perspective on how knowledge can be generated through research

Participants: people who form the sample in qualitative research

PICO question: formats used to help to create a search question in relation to a particular clinical issue in which P = population; I = Intervention; C = comparison; O = outcome

Positivism: a belief that reality is ordered, regular, can be studied objectively and quantified

Proportional stratified sampling: a form of sampling used in quantitative research to ensure subgroups (e.g. age, ethnicity, etc) within a population are present in a sample in the same proportions

Propositional knowledge: public knowledge usually given a formal status by its inclusion in educational programmes

Prospective studies: where data are collected in relation to a specific independent variable and the dependent variable is measured at a later date

Publication bias: the tendency to publish studies that report positive results resulting in a reported bias towards the effectiveness of a particular intervention

Non-propositional knowledge: personal knowledge linked to experience that is used by individuals to help them think and act

Reflection: the process by which someone actively considers an experience, critically appraising it in light of experience and knowledge, and develops a new perspective to be tested in new situations

Relevance: a consideration as to whether the findings from a study can be applied to a practice setting

Reliability: concerned with identifying if the results of a research study are dependable and replicable

Retrospective studies: research in which data are collected after an event of interest – for example, patients' notes may be examined for information in relation to a specific treatment and recovery

Rich (or thick) description: a term used in qualitative research meaning to give a full and thorough account of the research context, the meanings people attach to their experiences, their interpretation of issues, and what motivates them to behave/respond in particular ways

Rigour: ensuring that research is of a high quality, conducted in an appropriate way, and consistent with the underpinning philosophical principles

Sampling units: people who form the sample within quantitative research, sometimes known as subjects

Science: a body of knowledge, based on observation, experiment and measurement, organized in a systematic manner

Search engine: an electronic device which enables you to search the World Wide Web for information

Search filter: information put into the database to find the sources of evidence required

Secondary research: research using data from primary research rather than from an original source

Service evaluation: a systematic approach to gaining insight into patient satisfaction with services

Subjects: people who form the sample within quantitative research, sometimes known as sampling units

Systematic review: a rigorous review of research findings in relation to a specific clinical question

Tacit knowledge: knowledge well known to practitioners but not evident within the research-based literature

Tenacity: a source of knowledge believed simply because it has always been held as the truth

Thick or rich description: a term used in qualitative research meaning to give a full and thorough account of the research context, the meanings people attach to their experiences, their interpretation of issues, and what motivates them to behave/respond in particular ways

Transferability: a term used in qualitative research to describe the tentative application of research findings from one study to other similar groups of participants

Triangulation: an approach used in qualitative research to increase the rigor of the findings – entails considering the phenomenon of interest from different angles, usually in terms of its data, methodology, investigators, and theoretical framework

Trustworthiness: whether data from a research study can be considered dependable and credible

Validity: whether or not the claims made in a research study are accurate

Variables: a factor or trait that is likely to vary from one person/situation to another, such as weight, temperature, pain, and personality traits

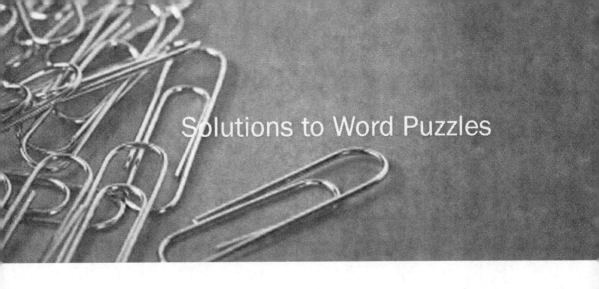

Solutions to Word Puzzles

Solution to Part 1 Crossword

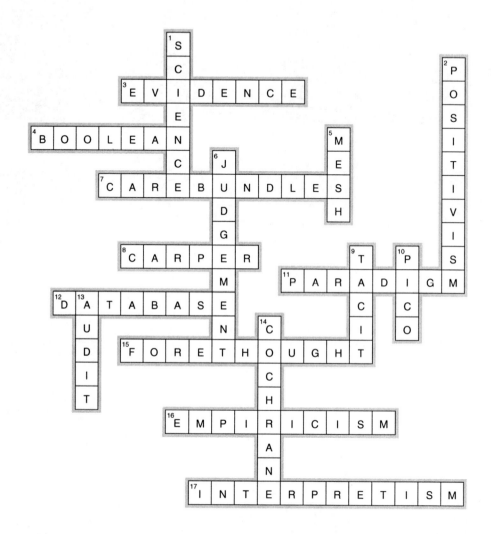

Solution to Part 2 Word Search

Hidden words

VALIDITY; RELIABILITY; TRUSTWORTHINESS; CREDIBILITY; DEPEND-
ABILITY; COMFIRMABILITY; TRANSFERABILITY; RIGOUR; VARIABLE;
HYPOTHESIS; PROBABILITY; STRATIFIED; ETIC; EMIC; BRACKETING;
META ANALYSIS; RELATIVE RISK; RANDOMISED; CONTROL; TRAIL;
PARAMETRIC; SNOWBALL; MEAN; MODE.

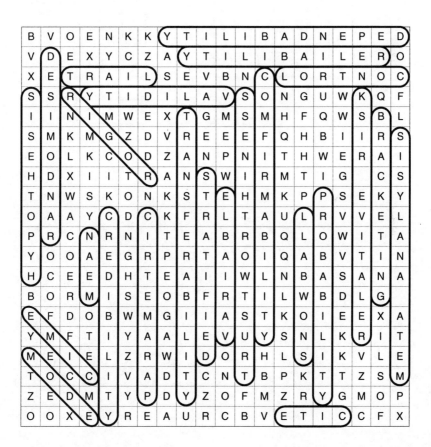

Solution to Part 3 Crossword

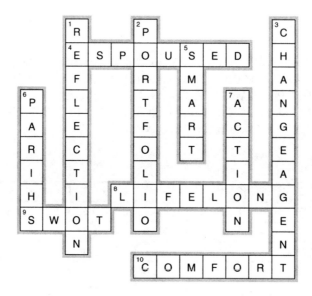

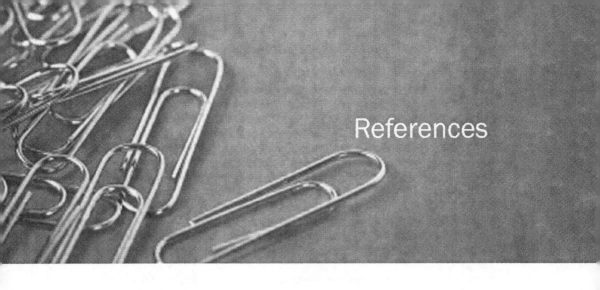

References

Akerman, L. (1997) 'Development, transition or transformation?: The question of change in organisations', in V. Iles and K. Sutherland (eds), *Organisational Change. National Co-ordinating Centre for NHS Service Delivery and Organisations*. London: R & D.

Akobeng, A.K. (2005) 'Understanding systematic reviews and meta-analysis'. Available at: www.adc.bmj.com (accessed August 2008).

Altman, D.G., Schulz, K.F., Moher, D., Egger, M., Davidoff, F., Elbourne, D., Gotzsche, P.C. and Lang, T. (2001) 'The revised CONSORT statement for reporting randomized trials: Explanation and elaboration', *Annals of Internal Medicine*. 134(8): 663–94.

Appraisal of Guidelines for Research and Evaluation Collaboration (AGREE) (2001) Appraisal of Guidelines for Research and Evaluation Instrument. Available at: www.agreecollaboration. org (accessed May 2008).

Avis, M. (1994) 'Reading research critically. 1. An introduction to appraisal: Designs and objectives', *Journal of Clinical Nursing*, 3: 227–34.

Bakalis, N. (2006) 'Clinical decision making in cardiac nursing: A review of the literature', *Nursing Standard*, 21(120): 39–46.

Barker, J. and Rush, B. (2009) 'Rehabilitation and recovery' in Mallik, M. Hall, C. and Howard, D. (eds.) *Nursing Knowledge and Practice: A decision-making approach* (3rd edn). London: Elsevier.

Benner, P. (1984) *From Novice to Expert: Excellence and power in clinical nursing practice*. Menlo Park: Addison Wesley.

Benner, P., Tanner, C. and Chesla, C. (1996) *Expertise in Nursing Practice: Caring clinical judgement and ethics*. New York: Springer.

Billay, D., Myrick, F., Luhanga, F. and Yonge, O. (2007) 'A pragmatic view of intuitive knowledge in nursing practice', *Nursing Forum*, 42(3): 147–55.

Bond, M. and Holland, S. (1998) *Skills of Clinical Supervision for Nurses*. Buckingham: Open University Press.

Borton, T. (1970) *Reach, Touch and Teach*. New York: McGraw-Hill.

Boud, D., Keogh, R. and Walker, D. (1985) *Reflection: Turning Experience into Learning*. London: Kogan Page.

Brady, N. and Lewin, L. (2007) 'Evidence–based nursing: Bridging the gap between research and practice', *Journal of Pediatric Health Care*, 21(1): 53–6.

Bridges, W. (2003) *Making Transitions: Making the most of change*. London: Nicholas Brealey.

Brown, R.A. (1992) *Portfolio Development and Profiling for Nurses. Central Health Studies Series No. 3*. Lancaster: Quay Publishers.

Buckingham, J., Fisher, B. and Sandue, D. (2008) 'Introduction to EBM'. Available at: www. ebm.ualberta.cg (accessed April 2008).

Bugers, J., Bailey, J., Klazinga, N., van der Bij, A., Grot, R. and Fender, G. (2002) 'Inside guidelines: Comparative analysis of recommendations and evidence in diabetes guidelines from 13 countries', *Diabetes Care*, 25(11): 1933–39.

Butterworth, T., Fauger, J. and Burnard, P. (eds) (1998) *Clinical Supervision and Mentorship in Nursing* (2nd edn). London: Stanley Thornes.

Butz, A. (2007) 'Evidence-based practice in nursing: Bridging the gap between research and practice', *Journal of Pediatric Health Care*, 21: 53–6.

Carper, B. (1978) 'Fundamentals patterns of knowing in nursing', *Advances in Nursing Science*, 1: 13–23.

Chinn, P.L. and Kramer, M.K. (2004) *Theory and Nursing: Integrated Knowledge Development* (6th edn). St Louis: C.V. Mosby.

Claxton, G. (1999) *Wise Up: The challenge of lifelong learning*. London: Bloomsbury.

Cochrane, A. (1972) *Effectiveness and Efficiency: Random Reflections on the NHS*. Abingdon: Burgess.

Colaizzi, P.F. (1978) 'Psychological research as the phenomenologists view it', in R. Valle and M. King, (eds), *Existential Phenomenological Alternative for Psychology*. Oxford: OUP, pp. 48–71.

Command Paper, CM 5207s (2001) *Learning from Bristol: The Report of the Public Inquiry into Children's Heart Surgery at the Bristol Royal Infirmary 1984–1995*. London: Department of Health.

Cormack, D.F.S. (ed.) (1996) *The Research Process in Nursing* (3rd edn). Oxford: Blackwell.

Craig, J.V. and Pearson, M. (2007) 'Evidence-based practice in nursing', in J.V. Craig and R.L. Smyth (eds), *The Evidence-Based Practice Manual for Nurses* (2nd edn). Edinburgh: Churchill Livingstone/Elsevier.

Cranston, M. (2002) 'Clinical effectiveness and evidence-based practice', *Nursing Standard*, 16(24): 39–43.

Cullum, N., Ciliska, D., Marks, S. and Haynes, B. (2008) 'An introduction to evidence-based nursing', in N. Cullum, D. Ciliska, S. Marks and B. Haynes (eds), *Evidence–Based Nursing: An introduction*. Oxford: Blackwell.

Dale, A.E. (2005) 'Evidence-based practice: Compatibility with nursing', *Nursing Standard*, 19(40): 48–53.

D'Auria, J. (2007) 'Using an evidence-based approach to critical appraisal', *Journal of Pediatric Health Care*, 21(5): 343–46.

Denzin, N.K. (1989) *The Research Act: A theoretical introduction to sociological methods*. Englewood Cliffs, NJ: Prentice-Hall.

Department of Health (DoH) (1997) *The New NHS: Modern and Dependable*. London: HMSO.

Department of Health (DoH) (1998) *A First Class Service: Quality in the New NHS*. London: HMSO.

Department of Health (DoH) (2001) *Research Governance Framework for Health and Social Care*. London: The Stationery Office.

Department of Health (DoH) (2003) *Building on the Best: Choice, Responsiveness and Equity in the NHS*. London: The Stationery Office.

Department of Health (DoH) (2005) *Research Governance Framework for Health and Social Care* (2nd edn). London: The Stationery Office.

Department of Health (DoH) (2006) *Agenda for change*. London: The Stationery Office.

DiCenso, A., Cullum, N. and Ciliska, D. (2008) 'Implementing evidence-based nursing: Some misconceptions', in N. Cullum, D. Ciliska, S. Marks and B. Haynes (eds), *Evidence-Based Nursing: An Introduction*. Oxford: Blackwell.

Doherty, C. and Doherty, W. (2005) 'Patient preferences for involvement in clinical decision-making within their secondary care and the factors that influence their preferences', *Journal of Nursing Management*, 13: 119–27.

Duffy, A. (2008) 'Guided reflection: A discussion of the essential components', *British Journal of Nursing*, 17(5): 334–39.

Edwards, S. (2002) 'Nursing knowledge: Defining new boundaries', *Nursing Standard*, 17(2): 40–4.

Eraut, M. (2000) 'Non-formal learning and tacit knowledge in professional work', *British Journal of Educational Psychology*, 70: 113–36.

Evans, D. and Pearson, A. (2001) 'Systematic reviews of qualitative research', *Clinical Effectiveness in Nursing*, 5: 111–19.

Ferguson, L.M. and Day, R.A. (2007) 'Challenges for new nurses in evidence-based practice', *Journal of Nursing Management*, 15: 107–13.

Field, N.J. and Lohr, K.N. (1990) *Clinical Practice Guidelines: Directions for a new programme*. Washington DC: Institute of Medicine.

Fitzpatrick, J. (2007) 'Finding the research for evidence-based practice: Part Two – Selecting the evidence', *Nursing Times*, 103(18): 32–3.

Finlayson, K. and Dixon, A. (2008) 'Qualitative meta-synthesis: A guide for the novice', *Nurse Researcher*, 15(2): 59–71.

Fleming, K. and Cullum, N. (1997) 'Doing the right thing', *Nursing Standard*, 12: 28–30.

Foster, N., Barlas, P., Chesterton, L. and Wong, J. (2001) 'Critical Appraisal Topics (CATs)', *Physiotherapy*, 87(4): 179–90.

Foucault, M. (1979) *The History of Sexuality*, Vol. 1. London: Penguin.

French, B. (2005) 'Evaluating research for use in practice: What criteria do specialist nurses use?', *Journal of Advanced Nursing*, 50(3): 235–43.

French, P. (1999) 'The development of evidence-based nursing', *Journal of Advanced Nursing*, 29(1): 72–8.

Fulbrook, P. and Mooney, S. (2003) 'Care bundles in critical care: A practice approach to evidence based practice', *Nursing in Critical Care*, 8(6): 249–55.

Gibbs, G. (1988) *Learning by Doing: A Guide to Teaching and Learning Methods*. London: FEU.

Glaser, B. and Strauss, A. (1967) *The Discovery of Grounded Theory*. Chicago, IL: Aldine.

Glasziou, P. and Haynes, B. (2005) 'The path from research to improved health outcomes', *Evidence-Based Nursing*, 8(2): 36–8.

Grant, G. and Ramcharan, P. (2006) 'User involvement in research', in K. Gerrish and A. Lacey (eds), *The Research Process in Nursing*. (5th edn). Oxford: Blackwell.

Greenhalgh, T. (2006) *How to Read a Paper: The basics of evidence-based medicine* (3rd edn). Oxford: Blackwell.

Greenhalgh, T., Robert, G., Macfarlane, F., Bate, P. and Kyriakidou, O. (2004) 'Diffusion of innovations in service organisations: systematic literature review and recommendations for future research', *Milbank Q*, 82: 581–629.

Greenhalgh, T. and Russell, J. (2006) 'Promoting the skills of knowledge translation in an online Master of Science course in primary health care', *Journal of Continuing Education in the Health Professions*, 26(2): 100–108.

Grol, R. and Grimshaw, J. (2003) 'From best evidence to best practice: effective implementation of change in patients' care', *The Lancet*, 362: 1225–30.

Guba, E. and Lincoln, Y. (1994) 'Competing paradigms in qualitative research', in N. Denzin and Y. Lincoln (eds), *Handbook of Qualitative Research*. London: Sage. pp. 105–117.

Gustafsson, C. and Fagerberg, I. (2004) 'Reflection, the way to professional development?', *Journal of Clinical Nursing*, 13: 271–80.

Haas, J.P. and Larson, E.L. (2008) 'Compliance with hand hygiene guidelines: Where are we in 2008?', *American Journal of Nursing*, 108(8): 40–4.

Harbison, J. (2006) 'Clinical judgement in the interpretation of evidence: A Bayesian approach', *Journal of Clinical Nursing*, 15: 1489–97.

Haynes, R.B. (2008) 'Of studies, summaries, synopses and systems: The "4S" evolution of services for finding current best evidence', in N. Cullum, D. Ciliska, R.B. Haynes and S. Marks (eds), *Evidence-Based Nursing*. Oxford: Blackwell.

Hewitt-Taylor, J. (2003) 'Reviewing evidence', *Intensive and Critical Care Nursing*, 19: 43–9.

Higgs, J. and Jones, M. (eds) (2000) 'Will evidence-based practice take the reasoning out of practice', in *Clinical Reasoning in the Health Professions* (2nd edn). Oxford: Butterworth Heineman.

Hull, C., Redfern, L. and Shuttleworth, A. (2005) *Profiles and Portfolios: A Guide for Health & Social Care* (2nd edn). Basingstoke: Palgrave MacMillan.

Hunt, J.M. (1996) 'Guest editorial', *Journal of Advanced Nursing*, 23: 423–5.

Huntington, A.D. and Gilmour, J.A. (2001) 'Rethinking representations, rewriting nursing texts: possibilities through feminism and Foucauldian thought', *Journal of Advanced Nursing*, 35(6): 902–8.

Iles, V. and Cranfield, S. (2004) Managing Change in the NHS. Developing Change Management Skills. A resource for health care professionals. National Co-ordinating Centre for NHS Service Delivery and Organisation, London. Available at: http://www.sdo.nihr.ac.uk/managingchange.html

Iles, V. and Sutherland, K. (2001) 'Managing Change in the NHS. Organisational Change: A review for health care managers, professionals and researchers'. National Co-ordinating Centre for NHS Service Delivery and Organisation, London. Available at: http://www.sdo.nihr.ac.uk/managingchange.html.

Ingersoll, G.L. (2000) 'Evidence-based nursing: What it is and what it isn't', *Nursing Outlook*, 48: 151–2.

Jarvis, P. (1992) 'Reflective practice and nursing', *Nurse Education Today*, 12: 174–81.

Jasper, M. (2003) *Beginning Reflective Practice*. Cheltenham: Nelson Thornes.

John, C. (2006) *Engaging Reflection in Practice: A Narrative Approach*. Oxford: Blackwell.

Kelly, D. and Connor, D. (1979) 'The emotional cycle of change', in J. Jones and J. Pfeiffer (eds), *The Annual Handbook for Group Facilitators*. Lajolla, CA: University Associates.

Kerliger, F.N. (1973) *Foundations of Behavioural Research* (2nd edn). New York: Holt, Reinhart and Winston.

Khan, K.S., Kunz, R., Kleijnen, A. and Antes, G. (2003) *Systematic Reviews to Support Evidence-Based Medicine*. London: The Royal Society of Medicine.

Kitson, A. (2002) 'Recognising relationships: Reflections on evidence-based practice', *Nursing Inquiry*, 9(3): 179–86.

Knowles, M. (1990) *The Adult Learner, A Neglected Species*. Houston, TX: Gulf.

Kolb, D. (1984) *Experiential Learning: Experience as the sources of learning and development*. New York: Prentice-Hall.

Kuhn, T. (1970) *The Structure of Scientific Revolution* (2nd edn). Chicago: University of Chicago Press.

Lancaster, J. and Lancaster, W. (eds) (1982) *Concepts for Advanced Nursing: The nurse as a change agent*. St Louis, IL: Mosby.

Lasater, K. (2006) 'Clinical judgement developing: Using simulation to create an assessment rubric', *Journal of Nurse Education*, 46(11): 496–503.

Leeman, J., Baernholdt, M. and Sandelowski, M. (2007) 'Developing a theory-based taxonomy of methods for implementing change in practice', *Journal of Advanced Nursing*, 58(2): 191–200.

Leininger, M.M. (1985) *Qualitative Research Methods in Nursing*. Orlando, FL: Grune & Straton.

Lewin, K. (1951) *Field Theory in Social Sciences*. New York: Harper & Row.

Lincoln, Y. and Guba, E.G. (1985) *Naturalistic Inquiry*. Newbury Park: Sage.

Lloyd Jones, M. (2005) 'Role development and effective practice in specialist and advanced practice in acute hospital settings: Systematic review and meta synthesis', *Journal of Advanced Nursing*, 49(2): 191–209.

MacGuire, J.M. (1990) 'Putting nursing research findings into practice: Research utilization as an aspect of the management of change', *Journal of Advanced Nursing*, 15: 614–20.

Manley, K., Hardy, S., Titchen, A., Garbett, R. and McCormack, B. (2005) *Changing Patients' Worlds through Nursing Expertise*. London: RCN.

Mantzoukas, S. (2007) 'A review of evidence-based practice, nursing research and reflection: Levelling the hierarchy', *Journal of Clinical Nursing*, 17: 214–23.

Mason, T. and Whitehead, E. (2003) *Thinking Nursing*. Buckingham: Open University Press.

McMullan, M., Endacott, R., Gray, M.A., Jasper, M., Miller, C.M.L., Scoles, J. and Webb, C. (2003) 'Portfolios and assessment of competency: a review of literature', *Journal of Advanced Nursing*, 41(3): 283–94.

McPhail, G. (1997) 'Management of change: An essential skill for nursing in the 1990s', *Journal of Nursing Management*, 5: 199–205.

Melnyk, B.M. and Fineout-Overholt, E. (2005) *Evidence-Based Practice in Nursing and Healthcare*. Philadelphia: Lippincott Williams & Wilkins.

Metz, A.J.R., Blasé, K. and Bowie, L. (2007) 'Implementing evidence-based practices: Six drivers of success. Brief Research-to-Results', *Child Trends,* October. Available at: www.child trends.org

Miller, S.A. and Forrest, J.J. (2001) 'Enhancing your practice decision making: PICO, good questions', *Journal of Evidence-Based Dental Practice*, 1: 136–41.

Moher, D., Cook, D.J., Eastwood, S., Olkin, I., Drummond, R. and Stroup, D.F. (1999) 'Improving the quality of reports of meta-analyses of randomised controlled trials: the QUOROM statement', *The Lancet,* 354: 1896–1900.

Mulhall, A. and Le May, A. (2001) *Taking Action: Moving Towards Evidence-Based Practice*. London: The Foundation of Nursing Studies.

National Research Ethics Service (2007) *Defining Research*. Available at: www.nres.npsa. nhs.uk (accessed January 2008).

NHS Institute for Innovation & Improvement (2005) 'Improvement Leaders' Guide. Managing the human dimensions of change. Personal and organisational development. Available at: www.institute.nhs.uk/improvementleadersguides

NHS Institute for Innovation & Improvement (2007) 'Improvement Leaders' Guide. Sustainability and its relationship with spread and adoption. General Improvement skills.' Available at: www.institute.nhs.uk/improvementleadersguides

Nickols, F. (2000) Change Management 101: A Primer. Available at: http:home.att.net/~ nickols/change.htm (accessed April 2003).

Nieswiadomy, R.M. (2008) *Foundations of Nursing Research* (5th edn). New Jersey: Pearson.

NMC (2002) *Supporting Nurses and Midwives through Lifelong Learning*. London: NMC.

NMC (2008) *Code of Conduct*. London: NMC.

Ochieng, B.M.N. (1999) 'Use of reflective practice in introducing change on the management of pain in a paediatric setting', *Journal of Nursing Management*, 7: 113–118.

O'Connor, A.M., Llewellyn-Thomas, H.A. and Flood, A.B. (2004) 'Modifying unwarranted variations in health care: Shared decision making using patient decision tools', *Health Affairs*, 63: 1–10.

Page, S. and Meerabeau, L. (2000) 'Achieving change through reflective practice: Closing the loop', *Nurse Education Today*, 20: 365–72.

Parahoo, K. (1997) *Nursing Research: Principles, process and issues* London: MacMillan.

Parahoo, K. (2006) *Nursing Research: Principles process and issues* (2nd edn). Basingstoke: Palgrave MacMillan.

Parkes, J., Hyde, C., Deeks, J. and Milne, R. (2001) 'Teaching critical appraisal skills in healthcare settings', *Cochrane Database of Systematic Reviews*, Issue 3.

Peile, E. (2004) 'Reflections from medical practice: Balancing evidence-based practice with practice-based evidence' in G. Thomas and R. Pring (eds), *Evidence-Based Practice in Education*. Berkshire: Open University Press.

Pearson, A., Field, J. and Jordan, Z. (2007) *Evidence-Based Clinical Practice in Nursing and Health Care*. Oxford: Blackwell.

Petticrew, M. and Roberts, H. (2003) 'Evidence, hierarchies and typologies: Horses for courses', *Journal of Epidemiology and Community Health*, 57: 527–29.

Pettigrew, A., Ferlie, E. and McFee, L. (1992) *Shaping Strategic Change*. London: Sage.

Polit, D.F. and Beck, C.T. (2008) *Nursing Research: Generating and Assessing Evidence for Nursing Practice* (8th edn). Philadelphia: Lippincott Williams & Wilkins.

Polit, D.F. and Hungler, B.P. (1989) *Essential of Nursing Research: Methods, Appraisal and Utilization* (2nd edn). Philadelphia: Lippincott.

Pollock, C., Grime, J., Baker, E. and Mantala, K. (2004) 'Meeting the information needs of psychiatric patients: Staff and patient perspectives', *Journal of Mental Health*, 13(4): 389–401.

Portney, L. (2004) 'Evidence-based practice and clinical decision making: It's not just the research course anymore', *Journal of Physical Therapy Education*, 18(3): 46–51.

Rolfe, G., Freshwater, D. and Jasper, M. (2001) *Critical Reflection for Nursing and the Helping Professions: A User's Guide*. Hampshire: Palgrave.

Royal College of Nursing (1996) *The Royal College of Nursing Clinical Effectiveness Intiative. A Strategic Framework*. London: RCN.

Rycroft-Malone, J. (2002) 'Getting evidence into practice: Ingredients for change', *Nursing Standard*, 16(37): 38–43.

Rycroft-Malone, J. (2004) 'The PARIHS Framework – a framework for guiding the implementation of evidence-based practice', *Journal of Nursing Care Quality*, 19(4): 297–304.

Rycroft-Malone, J., Harvey, G., Kitson, A., McCormack, D., Seers, K. and Titchen, A. (2002) 'Getting evidence into practice: Ingredients for change', *Nursing Standard*, 16(37): 38–43.

Rycroft-Malone, J., Seers, K., Titchen, A., Harvey, G., Kitson, A. and McCormack, B. (2004a) 'What counts as evidence in evidence-based practice?', *Journal of Advanced Nursing*, 47(1): 81–90.

Rycroft-Malone, J., Harvey, G., Seers, K., Kitson, A., McCormack, B. and Titchen, A. (2004b) 'An exploration of the factors that influence the implementation of evidence into practice', *Journal of Clinical Nursing*, 13(8): 913–24.

Sackett, D.L. (2008) 'The need for EMB. Collated PowerPoint Presentations'. Center for Evidence Based Evidence. Available at: http://www.cebm.net/index.aspx?o=1083

Sackett, D.L., Rosenberg, W.M.C., Grey, J.A.M., Haynes, R.B. and Richardson, W.S. (1996) 'Evidence based medicine: what it is and what it isn't. It's about integrating individual clinical expertise and the best external evidence', *British Medical Journal*, 312(7023): 71–2.

Sackett, D.L., Straus, S.E., Scott Richardson, W., Rosenberg, W.M.C., Grey, J.A.M. and Haynes, R.B. (2000) *Evidence-Based Medicine: How to practice and teach EBM*. London: Churchill Livingstone.

Sanderlin, B.W. and AbdulRahim, N. (2007) 'Evidence-based medicine, Part 6: An introduction to critical appraisal of clinical practice guidelines', JAOA, 107(8): 321–4.

Schon, D. (1983) *The Reflective Practitioner: How professionals think in action*. New York: Basic.

Schon, D. (1987) *Educating the Reflective Practitioner*. San Francisco, CA: Jossey-Bass.

Scott, S.D., Estabrooks, C.A., Allen, M. and Pollock, C. (2008) 'A context of uncertainty: How context shapes nurses' research utilization behaviours', *Qualitative Health Research*, 18(3): 347–57.

Shanley, C. (2007) 'Management of change for nurses: Lessons from the discipline of organizational studies', *Journal of Nursing Management*, 15: 538–46.

Sidani, S. (2006) 'Eliciting patient treatment preference: A strategy to integrate evidence-based and patient centered care: worldviews on evidence-based nursing', *Third Quarter*, 116–23.

Spenceley, S.M., O'Leary, K.A., Chizawsky, L.L.K., Ross, A.J. and Estabrooks, C.A. (2008) 'Sources of information used by nurses to inform practice: An integrative review', *International Journal of Nursing Studies*, 45: 954–70.

Spezial, H.J.S. and Carpenter, D.R. (2007) *Qualitative Research in Nursing* (4th edn). Philadelphia: Lippincott Williams & Wilkins.

Stevens, K.R. (2004) 'ACE Star Model of EBP: Knowledge translation'. Academic Centre for Evidence-Based Practice, the University of Texas Health Science Center at San Antonio. Available at: www.acestar.uthscsa.edu (accessed May 2008).

Stott, R. (1999) 'Citation pearl growing'. Available at: http://newadonis.creighton.edu/HSL/searching/PearlGrowing.html (accessed August 2008).

Strauss, A. and Corbin, J. (1990) *Basics of Qualitative Research: Grounded theory, procedures and techniques*. Thousand Oaks, CA: Sage.

Tanner, C.A. (2006) 'Thinking like a nurse: A research-based model of clinical judgement in nursing', *Journal of Nurse Education*, 45(6): 204–11.

Tarlier, D. (2004) 'Mediating the meaning of evidence through epistemological diversity', *Nursing Inquiry*, 12(2): 126–34.

Thomas, G. (2004) 'Introduction: evidence and practice', in G. Thomas and R. Pring (eds), *Evidence-Based Practice in Education*. Berkshire: Open University Press.

Thompson, C., McCaughan, D., Cullun, N., Sheldon, T., Thompson, D, and Mulhall, A. (2002) 'Nurses' use of research information in clinical decision making: A descriptive and analytical study: final report'. NHS R&D Programme In Evaluation Methods.

Thompson, C. (2003) 'Clinical experience as evidence in evidence-based practice', *Journal of Advanced Nursing*, 43(3): 230–7.

Thompson, D.S., Moore, K.N. and Estabrooks, C.A. (2008) 'Increasing research use in nursing: Implications for clinical educators and managers', *Evidence Based Nursing*, 11: 35–9.

Titchin, A. and Higgs, J. (eds) (2001) *Professional Practice in Health Education and the Creative Arts*. Oxford: Blackwell.

Timmins, F. (2008) *Making Sense of Portfolios: A guide for nursing students*. Berkshire: Open University Press.

Tingle, J. (2002) 'Mental health nurses: Changing practice?', *Journal of Clinical Nursing*, 11(5): 657–63.

UKCC (1995) *PREP and You: Maintaining your registration*. London: UKCC.

Upshur, R.E.G., Van Den Kerkhof, E.G. and Goel, V. (2001) 'Meaning and measurement: An inclusive model of evidence in health care', *Journal of Evaluation in Clinical Practice* 7(2): 91–6.

Upton, T. and Brooks, B. (1995) *Managing Change in the NHS*. London: Kogan Page.

White, J. (1995) 'Patterns of knowing: Review, critique and update', *Advances in Nursing Science*, 17(4): 73–86.

Williams, J. (2001) 'Using reflection in everyday orthopaedic nursing practice', *Journal of Orthopaedic Nursing*. 10(1): 49–55.

World Medical Association (2004) Declaration of Helsinki. Ethical Principles for Medical Research Involving Human Subjects. http://www.wma.net/e/policy/b3.htm

Zellner, K., Boerst, C.J. and Tabb, W. (2007) 'Statistics used in current nursing research', *Journal of Nurse Education*, 46(2): 55–9.

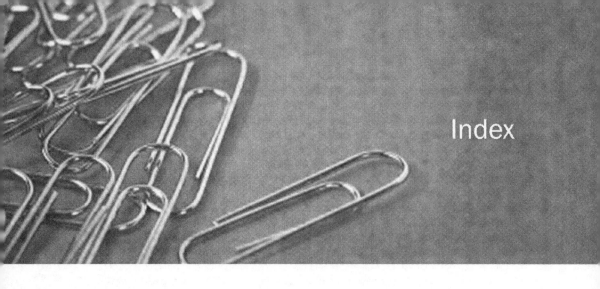

Index

This index is in word-by-word order. Page references in *italics* indicate figures, those in **bold** indicate tables

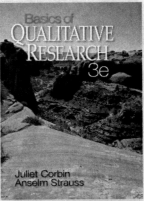
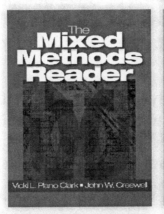
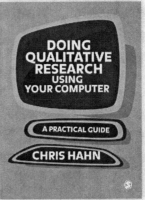
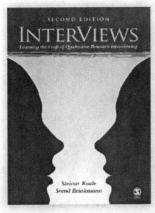
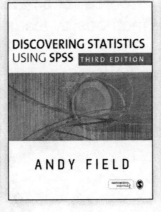
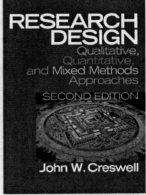
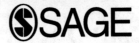

Supporting researchers for more than forty years

Research methods have always been at the core of SAGE's publishing. Sara Miller McCune founded SAGE in 1965 and soon after she published SAGE's first methods book, *Public Policy Evaluation*. A few years later, she launched the Quantitative Applications in the Social Sciences series – affectionately known as the 'little green books'.

Always at the forefront of developing and supporting new approaches in methods, SAGE published early groundbreaking texts and journals in the fields of qualitative methods and evaluation.

Today, more than forty years and two million little green books later, SAGE continues to push the boundaries with a growing list of more than 1,200 research methods books, journals, and reference works across the social, behavioural, and health sciences.

From qualitative, quantitative and mixed methods to evaluation, SAGE is the essential resource for academics and practitioners looking for the latest in methods by leading scholars.

www.sagepublications.com

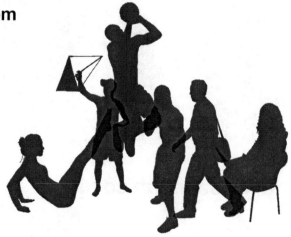

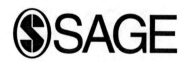